Examinations in Medicine

P. R. Fleming, M.D., F.R.C.P.
Senior Lecturer in Medicine, Westminster Medical School.

P. H. Sanderson, M.B., F.R.C.P.
Reader in Medicine, St. Mary's Hospital Medical School.

J. F. Stokes, M.D., F.R.C.P., F.R.C.P.(E.)
Physician, University College Hospital.

H. J. Walton, M.D., F.R.C.P.(E.), F.R.C.Psych.
Professor of Psychiatry, University of Edinburgh.

Foreword by
G.A. Smart, M.D., F.R.C.P.
Director, British Postgraduate Medical Federation.

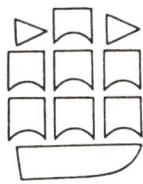 John Sauire Medical Library

CHURCHILL LIVINGSTONE
Edinburgh London and New York 1976

CHURCHILL LIVINGSTONE

Medical Division of Longman Group Limited
Distributed in the United States of America by
Longman Inc., 72 Fifth Avenue, New York, N.Y. 10011
and by associated companies, branches and
representatives throughout the world.

© Longman Group Limited, 1976

*All rights reserved. No part of this publication may
be reproduced, stored in a retrieval system or
transmitted in any form or by any means, electronic,
mechanical, photocopying, recording or otherwise,
without the prior permission of the publishers
(Churchill Livingstone, 23 Ravelston Terrace, Edinburgh)*

ISBN 0 443 01408 6

Middlesex HA1 3UJ

Acc. No............ Class............

Printed in Hong Kong

Foreword

So many of us have suffered from examinations during our childhood and the earlier part of our adult life that the very memory may be associated with a recurrence of those psychosomatic phenomena such as 'examination halitosis' which all but a few of us, including the most relaxed and the kindliest, must have experienced, and, later, observed. Traditionally, examinations have been feared because so much hung on the result - and yet careful scrutiny of the traditional examination techniques used in medicine has shown that luck must inevitably play a crucial part in the outcome. Quite clearly the average examinee believes that it is to a large extent a game of chance - that it is quite impossible for anyone to know all that he might be asked and that therefore if only his luck should hold he might somehow or other defeat the examiners and bluff his way through to victory.

But this is not what examinations are all about - or at least it ought not to be. A candidate who is fully prepared and up to standard ought confidently to pass. The trouble is that so much of the process has hitherto been intuitive and arbitrary. Thus has grown the movement to reject examinations entirely, replacing them, if by anything, by some process wherein supervisors give reports of satisfactory attendance and progress. But such reports can be just as arbitrary and subject to just as much human error as the traditional examination. Moreover, in a subject like medicine, where the passing of an examination after a prescribed training may confer legal rights of importance to people's lives, the public naturally demands that before this can occur certain minimum standards must be seen to have been attained. Hence the importance of improving the examination as an instrument which can determine standards and predict a satisfactory future performance to the maximum possible extent.

Examinations have other uses. They are a potent force in determining what a student learns and, if chance could be minimised so that an examination could be made to diagnose with a fair degree of accuracy a student's limitations and shortcomings, it would be most beneficial as an aid in making good those deficiencies. Examinations which are relevant and which are accurate in diagnosis and in assessing standards may also be used to make comparisons, not only between students, but between groups of students. Hence such examinations could be of great value to those professionally engaged in medical education as an aid to improving the efficiency of the methods used by them and by the institutions in which they work.

For all these reasons it is most important that a constant effort should be made to improve the relevance, the diagnostic (and if possible the prognostic) accuracy, and the reproducibility of examinations. The ideal examination would be of immense help to all concerned with the outcome - students, teacher and public alike, and such a 'perfect' examination would enable people to progress through their education and training at their own pace, rather than in a set time (set so that the slowest can only just cope) as at present. In principle there would be nothing to fear, if one is not afraid of the truth.

The authors of this handbook are to be congratulated on putting together the present position and in outlining the progress that has been made towards improving medical examinations in this country. Some aspects of examining, such as the multiple-choice technique, have become very sophisticated within their own limited sphere, and great efforts are needed to develop methods of equal validity to test other required attributes. A great debt is owing to the Nuffield Provincial Hospitals Trust for the support they gave to A.S.M.E. which enabled the Association to set up a Working Party to consider the feasibility of establishing a Central Examining Service in this country. For a number of reasons such a service has not yet come into being, but if it were a *service*, rather than a body which merely proposed to set national examinations, thereby tending to stultify educational experiments, it would be of immense value. One can only hope that the idea has not been buried forever and that (although this is not the purpose of the authors) the description in these pages of the progress which has so far been made in examination techniques in this country will serve to convince the reader that such a development is ultimately desirable.

G.A. Smart

Preface

The first inkling that this handbook might one day come to be written occurred in the course of an informal dinner held during the series of meetings of the Working Party set up in 1969 by the Association for the Study of Medical Education to look into the possibilities of some form of central medical examining service. If it did no more, this working party provided a forum for the exchange of ideas between many men interested in and concerned with evaluation; over the last few years some of these ideas have crystallised to form the basis of the chapters which follow.

This handbook is not intended to be a comprehensive account of examinations in medicine but more a practical guide which may be of assistance to those who are trying to make fairer, more reliable and more valid tests. The number of requests that some of us get for help in this field suggests that there is a need for guidance in Britain and the handbook has a frankly British orientation. It is also hoped that it may prove of use to those in the so-called developing countries who are at present engaged in modifying or evolving their own examinations at both undergraduate and postgraduate levels.

Though much of our experience derives from examining in internal medicine in general and in the MRCP in particular, this handbook is designed to have wider relevance. The needs of those entrusted with the responsible task of evaluation without the analytical help provided by a computer are recognised, and some time is spent in discussing ways in which the discriminatory power of questions can be calculated by hand.

The current and welcome move to use examinations, whenever possible, as an educational instrument does not imply that they are likely to disappear; indeed, new tests are being devised to measure the quality of foreign medical graduates who wish to come and make a career in Britain. When examinations are designed, it is important that they should be relevant and comprehensive. If they rely exclusively on the methods of assessment which are known to be reliable there is a danger that they may evaluate only some of the attributes desirable in a doctor. We need to remember the old Chinese proverb which tells us that if we look at a leopard through a narrow enough tube all we shall see is a spot; likewise if we look at a medical student only through the medium of a multiple choice question all we shall see is a fact.

This handbook gives an account of those instruments on

which we think we can rely with reasonable confidence. The
arguments set out apply to all disciplines, though the examples
given are mostly derived from clinical medicine. We have to
accept that some of our tools are still blunt and that the
development of techniques and criteria for medical audit and
the polishing of tests for the assessment of attitudes must
occupy much of our thought and energies for the future.

London and Edinburgh, 1975.   P.R.F.
                                                           P.H.S.
                                                           J.F.S.
                                                           H.J.W.

Contents

	Foreword	v
	Preface	vii
1	The Current Scene	1
2	The Content of Examinations and Examining Methods	4
3	Testing in the Cognitive Domain	11
4	Psychomotor Skills	29
5	Assessment of Professional Attitudes	39
6	Scoring	49
7	Analysis of Results	67
8	Organisation of Examinations	80
9	Progressive Assessment	89
10	A Look to the Future	95

Appendices

A	Significance of Correlation Coefficients for Varying Numbers of Observations	102
B	Determination and Significance of a Tetrachoric Correlation Coefficient	104
C	Combining Correlation Coefficients	107
D	Tests for Internal Reliability	108
E	Criteria for the Presentation of Projected Material	110
	Index	113

1. The Current Scene

The pattern of medical examinations in the United Kingdom took shape towards the end of the nineteenth century. This pattern - of written papers, orals and clinicals (or practicals) - has been modified in detail in the last twenty years or so but has been retained, in its essentials, by most examining bodies up to the present day. Before reviewing the current scene in more detail, it is salutary to study briefly the way in which this traditional system evolved.

The written papers have the longest pedigree having been introduced into Chinese medical examinations in the fifth century A.D. as a modification of the even older examinations for the mandarinate. They played no part, however, in European medical examinations until the eighteenth century at which time knowledge of Chinese customs was reaching Europe as a result of the writings of Jesuit missionaries. During the next hundred years they became widely used on the Continent; in Britain progress was rather slow but, by the middle of the nineteenth century, almost all British medical examining bodies were setting written papers.

The oral examination is derived directly from the mediaeval 'disputation' which for many years, from the thirteenth century onwards, was the main, if not the only, method of examination in medicine and in other disciplines. At times in the past the oral examination, designed to test a candidate's knowledge of the writings of the ancients, assumed the quasi-liturgical form mocked by Molière (Garrison, 1929); by the nineteenth century there was more spontaneity in the interrogation and the contemporary 'viva' differs little from the form it assumed over a century ago.

In comparison with the other parts of medical examinations the 'clinical' is an innovation. Although regarded by some with disfavour when the idea was first mooted in the mid-nineteenth century, the 'clinical' rapidly became part of all examinations in the clinical disciplines and was made compulsory, in qualifying examinations, by the General Medical Council in 1882. Like the 'viva', it remains unchanged from its original form to this day.

UNDERGRADUATE EXAMINATIONS

Two clear purposes underlie the series of examinations taken during and at the end of the undergraduate medical course. The first is to identify those candidates worthy of the degree or diploma awarded by the examining institution. This process of graduation is inextricably linked with the second purpose - the recognition of the new graduate as licensed to practise medicine. This aspect of 'finals' as a 'qualifying' examination stems from the need to ensure that the public is served by medical men and women of proven competence. This need has been felt by civilised communities for centuries and was formally recognised in Britain by the Medical Act of 1858. The importance which the medical profession attaches intuitively to this is illustrated by the fact that anxious medical students are much more likely to enquire whether one of their contemporaries has 'qualified' than whether he has 'graduated'.

The fact that the undergraduate courses and examination systems of many universities all lead to qualification and temporary registration implies that, despite all the demonstrable differences between examining bodies, there is a common 'core' of knowledge, skills and attitudes which should be possessed by all successful finals candidates. This is almost certainly the case although attempts to specify the nature of this 'core' precisely have been rare and none have commanded more than local acceptance. Few comparisons between different universities have been made, except by the somewhat dubious yardstick of the external examiner, although the Universities of Edinburgh, Liverpool and Newcastle have recently incorporated common material in their multiple-choice question papers (Ricketts *et al.*, 1974). No very striking difference between the undergraduates of the three medical schools emerged and such differences as there were could have been partly due to the fact that the examination was not taken in the same clinical year in all three universities. Nevertheless this study was extremely valuable if only as an example to others. The exchange of objective test material between universities might well, if the results were carefully analysed, lead ultimately to some agreement on the knowledge which should be possessed by newly qualified doctors.

Almost all the qualifying examinations in Britain are conducted by universities whose primary function is to teach. This is as it should be because it is now accepted that assessment is an important part of the educational process. Recognising this, many universities now make extensive use of progressive assessment, particularly in relation to qualities such as reliability and initiative which are difficult, if not impossible, to assess in traditional examinations. This is not to say that there is no place for examining bodies which have no teaching function, such as the Conjoint Board. If such organisations did not exist it would have been necessary to invent them if only to cater for those who, having studied medicine outside Britain, wish to obtain a qualification which entitles them to practise medicine in this country as the equals of British graduates.

POSTGRADUATE EXAMINATIONS

The concept of continuous assessment throughout a course of training cannot be easily applied in the postgraduate field. Attempts to do so have been made in America where candidates for postgraduate examinations are required to have undergone a course of training which is approved, as a whole, by the examining body. In Britain the policy has been to recognise individual posts, rather than courses, as suitable for training. As a result, there is little opportunity for co-ordinated progressive assessment. This deficiency is compensated, to some extent, by the greater flexibility of training programmes but it must be admitted that the dividing line between a flexible and a haphazard programme is a fine one.

Most British postgraduate diploma examinations can be taken about four years after graduation and all the Royal Colleges, with the exception of the Colleges of Physicians, specify in detail the postgraduate experience which is required before entry to the examination is accepted. Thus the majority of British postgraduate diplomas imply that the holder is ready to enter specialist training, usually at senior registrar level. In Britain we have set our faces against the idea of an 'exit' examination, in contrast to the extensive system of Board examinations provided at the end of specialist training in the U.S.A.. No one who has studied the pages of the Medical Directory could imagine that the British have a natural antipathy to postgraduate diplomas. There is general recognition in Britain that it is not yet possible to assess in any quantifiable terms *all* the attributes of a fully-trained specialist. It is probable that postgraduate examinations are taken earlier here than in the United States.

REFERENCES

Garrison, F.H. (1929) *An Introduction to the History of Medicine*, 4th edition. Philadelphia and London: Saunders.
Ricketts, B.S., Anderson, J., Richmond, J., and Wood, W.A. (1974) Multiple choice questions in medicine: comparison of performances of M.B. candidates from three universities. *British Journal of Medical Education*, 8, 209.

2. The Content of Examinations and Examining Methods

Examinations are essentially measuring instruments by means of which the change in an individual's behaviour produced by an educational process can be assessed. The term 'change of behaviour' may jar on some readers by reason of its unfamiliarity but they may perhaps be persuaded that behaviour is the 'outward and visible sign' by which alone a student's knowledge and thought-processes can become manifest. A prerequisite for the design of a measuring instrument is a precise definition of what is to be measured; if, for example, the area of a geometrical figure is to be measured, a ruler will suffice if the figure is rectangular, whereas if it is irregular, a planimeter is required. Thus the nature of any examination is determined by the answers to two deceptively simple questions - 'What is to be tested?' and 'How is it to be tested?'.

THE CONTENT OF EXAMINATIONS

A detailed discussion of the first of these questions would involve consideration of the whole medical curriculum including the all-important preliminary definition of objectives. This subject has been discussed by numerous authors and will not be elaborated here. However, a few remarks, particularly relevant to examinations, may be in order. Syllabuses are published, by medical schools and other bodies, prescribing the subjects to be studied in the medical course. The detail contained within these syllabuses varies greatly, particularly between subjects. For example, in a pre-medical subject such as chemistry detailed specifications such as 'Velocity of chemical reactions; law of mass action; temperature coefficient...' may well appear. Syllabuses in medicine, on the other hand, frequently contain such general expressions as 'Instruction in the principles and practice of medicine'. Realising the deficiencies of traditional syllabuses, some organisations have published detailed accounts of their curricular objectives, often in behavioural terms. For example, the University of Illinois (1973) has published an account of their objectives in the basic medical sciences and clinical subjects, specifying precisely what is expected of the students at each stage of the course; this runs to several hundred pages. The Royal Australasian College of Surgeons has likewise defined the syllabus for its Primary Fellowship examination in great detail. In too many cases, however, in the absence of a detailed definition of objectives, the content of the

undergraduate course is determined by the pattern and scope
of the examinations. It is difficult to interest medical
students, at least in their final year, in subjects in which
they will be examined, at most, cursorily and it has not esc-
aped the attention of some specialists that the only way to
ensure sufficient attention to their subjects in the undergraduate course is to insist on a sizeable representation for
these subjects in the examinations. Of the postgraduate examining bodies, few, if any, publish a detailed syllabus of
study suitable for their clinical examinations. It is debatable whether such a publication would be desirable or even
feasible as very frequent revisions would be needed to allow
for today's rapidly changing medical practice. In any case,
it must be unusual for candidates to be quite unaware of what
is required of them although, possibly, candidates from overseas may be at some disadvantage in this respect.

In a widely-used classification, educational objectives,
in medicine as well as in other disciplines, are allotted to
three 'domains' - *cognitive, psychomotor* and *affective*. It is
convenient to use a similar classification when considering
the content of examinations. Thus, an examination should be
designed to answer three questions about each candidate as
follows: (i) 'What does he know?' (cognitive), (ii) 'What
can he do?' (psychomotor), (iii) 'What sort of person is he?'
(affective). The extent to which each of these attributes is
tested varies greatly with the subject. Thus, in an examination in Greek history, assessment of the candidates is in the
cognitive domain only and testing in the psychomotor and affective domains is not required. In a driving test, on the
other hand, testing of psychomotor skills is essential and,
in the cognitive domain, a few questions are asked on the High-
way Code; assessment in the affective domain is probably rarely
used, although one imagines that a tendency to swear at other
road-users might well impress an examiner unfavourably.

Within the cognitive domain educational objectives and hence
the attributes to be tested have been classified by Bloom *et al*,
(1956). Their taxonomy was designed to be applicable to any
discipline and has been modified specifically for medical examinations by Charvat, McGuire and Parsons (1968). This taxonomy
is referred to in later chapters as the CMP classification and
is as follows:
- (a) Knowledge of fundamental vocabulary, facts, concepts, principles, laws, methods and procedures
- (b) Understanding of these facts, concepts, etc
- (c) Ability to understand and interpret data
- (d) Ability to solve relevant problems
- (e) Judgement in evaluating a total situation
- (f) Ability to create a new synthesis.

The assessment of these attributes presents to examiners
a series of problems which become progressively more difficult
as one proceeds beyond knowledge and understanding of facts to

problem-solving and evaluation of a total situation. Many sophisticated and reliable techniques exist for testing factual knowledge; these are described in detail in Chapter 3 which also contains accounts of some, more or less successful, attempts to solve the problems of the assessment of higher attributes.

In practice, in medicine, written papers are concerned with the cognitive domain only and usually test at a rather low taxonomic level. The cognitive domain is also explored in the oral examination in which it is possible to test higher attributes; for example, a candidate's ability to interpret data and solve problems can be assessed. It must be admitted, however, that many of the questions asked in oral examinations are at the level of factual knowledge only. If it is accepted that there are other, better, ways of testing such knowledge, such oral questions are inappropriate as, of course, are similar questions which sometimes intrude into clinical examinations.

In medicine, testing in the psychomotor domain is concerned with the assessment of candidates' abilities in laboratory work, physical examination, operative surgery and the like. The problems involved are discussed in Chapter 4 but two general points concerning the relevance and feasibility of practical tests are worth emphasising here. The first concerns the testing of laboratory skills, particularly in undergraduate examinations. It is undeniable that practical work, for example in the basic medical sciences, plays an important part in deepening students' understanding of physiological and pharmacological concepts. It is open to question, however, whether it is appropriate to incorporate such practical work in an examination when there are better ways of assessing candidates' understanding. It seems more sensible to test the end-product of the educational process rather than the means by which that end-product has been obtained. The second point is related to the clinical disciplines. There is no argument, at least in the United Kingdom, about the importance of testing clinical skills. The problem here is one of feasibility. It is extremely difficult to design a realistic test of a candidate's skill as a clinical diagnostician, let alone as a practising surgeon. Many clinical examinations have been designed, in the past, in terms of their practicability rather than their suitability for the testing of the appropriate skills.

The greatest problems of all are presented by attempts to test in the affective domain - the assessment of attitudes, habits and values. The attributes to be tested in this area, listed by Charvat *et al.* (1968) are as follows:
- (a) Acceptance of responsibility for patient welfare
- (b) Concern and consideration for patient and patient's family
- (c) Recognition of medical capabilities and limitations
- (d) Ability to establish effective relationships with colleagues and other members of the health team
- (e) Regular observation of appropriate safeguards

(f) An inquiring mind
(g) Willingness to use medical capabilities to contribute to community as well as individual patient welfare.

A requirement to test all candidates in these respects in a final examination would be greeted by most examiners with dismay, not to say derision. Such attempts as are made at present are informal, wholly subjective and, probably, completely unreliable. They consist of an assessment of a candidate's demeanour in the thoroughly artificial atmosphere of the oral and clinical examinations and of his 'bedside manner' in the best sense of that term. Few examiners are wholly uninfluenced by these and some claim to rely quite heavily on their 'general impression' of the candidate. Most, however, realising that anxiety can manifest itself in many ways, are prepared to pardon unprepossessing behaviour and quite readily attribute it to the stress of the examination.

A more serious attempt to assess a candidate in the affective domain can be made if a programme of progressive assessment allows his examiners to study his behaviour over many weeks or months. Even with this longer acquaintance the informality and subjectivity of most assessments seriously impair their reliability. Progress has been made in this area, however, and current views are presented in Chapter 5.

THE TOOLS OF THE TRADE

Once the attributes which are to be tested have been precisely defined, it then becomes possible to choose or, if necessary, design suitable procedures for this purpose. At present examinations in medicine consist of a variable mixture of written papers in essay or multiple-choice format, practical and clinical examinations and orals. The merits and demerits of these procedures are discussed in subsequent chapters but some general points on the criteria by which they should be judged - as measuring instruments - will be made here. Two criteria in particular, *reliability* and *validity*, have been identified.

Reliability

This criterion refers to the requirement that independent assessments of a single personal attribute should yield identical results. A measuring instrument must, above all else, be consistent in its operation; an elastic ruler is of very limited value. On this score most methods of examining in medicine are seriously deficient, mainly on account of their lack of objectivity. Essay questions have been particularly criticised largely, we suspect, because it is easier to demonstrate low reliability in this area than in others. In medicine, Bull (1956) was one of the first to investigate this subject. He showed that the marks allotted by different examiners to the same set of essays correlated very poorly and, also, that the same examiner, marking the same paper on two separate occasions, produced two very different sets of marks. This work has been confirmed many times and Lennox (1967), for example, showed that it was possible for six separate examiners, marking a single essay, to award marks ranging from 'Fail' to 'Honours'. In extenuation he pointed out that the essay in question was a very good answer to a question somewhat different from the one which had been set.

Studies of oral and clinical examinations have yielded similar results (McGuire, 1966; Fleming *et al.*, 1974). This might have been expected by anyone who realises that an examiner, face to face with a candidate, is as likely as the next man to be influenced by his preconceptions and prejudices, however hard he tries to avoid it.

Various attempts have been made to increase the reliability and objectivity of medical examinations. Most examining bodies, realising that 'there is safety in numbers', arrange that a candidate's performances in different parts of an examination are assessed by as many examiners as possible; there is evidence that, on the whole, prejudices tend to cancel each other out. The close-marking system, in which marks are awarded over a very small range about the pass mark, is also an attempt to minimize the effect of examiner variability; this system has disadvantages, however, which are discussed in Chapter 6. Another useful measure is the feed-back to examiners of their marking habits compared with those of their colleagues. Complete objectivity has been achieved, in a limited part of the cognitive domain only, by the use of multiple-choice questions; a high degree of objectivity and reliability can also be obtained if the candidate's answers to questions can be confined to a very few words.

Several techniques exist for the formal measurement of reliability, although not all are applicable in routine practice. By the use of these techniques, which are described in Chapter 7, it is possible to determine the extent to which factors other than the candidate's ability determine the mark he obtains in an examination.

Validity

Validity has been subdivided into *content validity*, *predictive (criterion-related) validity* and *construct validity*. Content validity describes the extent to which an examination samples a candidate's knowledge, psychomotor skills or attitudes over the whole range of the subject being tested. On this score, as well as on that of reliability, essay questions are clearly inferior to multiple-choice questions by virtue of the number of topics which can be covered in a single examination paper. This does not imply that multiple-choice questions are necessarily valid; a low validity is often due to the questions being too easy or too difficult and thus failing to discriminate between candidates at the appropriate level.

The concept of content validity can be applied to other types of medical examinations. For example, a clinical examination is presumably intended to be a test of a candidate's ability to elicit and interpret points in a history and physical signs and to organise this information into a coherent set of clinical problems. The validity of such a test would be low if a candidate were allotted a nearly symptom-free patient with aortic incompetence and perceptive deafness as a long case, followed by short 'spot' cases with acromegaly, psoriasis of the finger-nails and hereditary haemorrhagic telangiectasia. Such a sequence could hardly be regarded as representing a fair sample of clinical medicine yet is by no means unlikely to occur in some clinical examinations. The construction of an examination of high content validity therefore demands careful matching of the content of the examination with the attributes which a successful candidate is required to possess.

Predictive validity is concerned with the extent to which an examination predicts future performance or yields results similar to those of another test of the same attributes. Thus it seems to have been agreed, in the past at any rate, that persons achieving a First in Greats have been successful in Civil Service careers. It can be said therefore that, however unlikely it might seem, Greats has a certain predictive validity for success as a Civil Servant. In medicine, one of us has published results showing high predictive validity of an end-of-course test for the results of a qualifying examination (Sanderson, 1973). Similar studies have been published on the relationship between the two parts of the MRCP (UK) examination. As Part I must be passed before a candidate is permitted to enter for Part II, it is important that Part I should have a high validity as a predictor of a candidate's performance in Part II (Study Group, 1967; Fleming *et al.*, 1974).

Construct validity refers to the type of intellectual activity required to pass the examination. Thus, if an examination were intended to be a test of problem-solving ability, it would be of low validity if the questions could be answered from memory alone. It may seem that this area overlaps somewhat with content validity; the situation may be clarified if content validity is regarded as being concerned with the range of a candidate's knowledge or expertise and construct validity with the depth of his understanding.

THE OBJECTIVE APPROACH

It must be admitted that examinations in medicine, and in most other disciplines, are deficient in many respects when subjected to a rigorous analysis. Fortunately, many examiners are now aware of these deficiencies and steps are being taken to improve the situation. Among these perhaps the most important are the attempts to increase the objectivity of medical examinations. No one would suggest that examiners should become automata but many examiners are now prepared to accept some constriction of their scope in the interests of more reliable and valid examinations. The objective approach is most familiar in the form of multiple-choice questions which test quite well in the cognitive domain, at least at the lower taxonomic levels. It is important to develop methods of assessment in the psychomotor and affective domains which approach the objectivity of multiple-choice questions.

REFERENCES

Bloom, B.S., Engelhart, M.D., Furst, E.J., Hill, W.H. and Krathwohl, D.R. (1956) *Taxonomy of Educational Objectives*. London : Longmans.

Bull, G.M. (1956) An Examination of the Final Examination in Medicine. *Lancet*, 2, 368.

Charvat, J., McGuire, C and Parsons, V. (1968) *A Review of the Nature and Uses of Examinations in Medical Education*. Geneva : World Health Organisation.

Fleming, P.R., Manderson, W.G., Matthews, M.B., Sanderson, P.H. and Stokes, J.F. (1974) Evolution of an Examination : M.R.C.P. (U.K.). *British Medical Journal*, 1, 99.

Lennox, B. (1967) Multiple Choice. *British Journal of Medical Education*, 1, 340.

McGuire, C. (1966) The Oral Examination as an Assessment of Professional Competence. *Journal of Medical Education*, 41, 274.

Sanderson, P.H. (1973) Prediction of Student Performance by Multiple Choice Testing. *British Journal of Medical Education*, 7, 251.

Study Group of the Royal College of Physicians of London (1967) Experience of Multiple-Choice-Question Examination for Part I of the M.R.C.P. *Lancet*, 2, 1034.

The University of Illinois College of Medicine (1973) *Curriculum Objectives*. London : British Medical Association.

3. Testing in the Cognitive Domain

MULTIPLE-CHOICE QUESTIONS

Of the techniques available for testing in this area, by far the best adapted to the requirements of objectivity and reliability is the multiple-choice question (MCQ) in its various forms. This device has in the past received almost idolatrous acclaim; more recently some examiners, as the results of much experience, have questioned its extensive use in medical examinations (Dudley, 1973). We would certainly not advocate the exclusive use of multiple-choice questions in cognitive testing, and reasons for this attitude will be set out below. At the same time few examiners would now like to abandon altogether such a powerful and versatile tool, which has acted as a potent stimulus in the move towards more objective testing.

The basic idea of the MCQ will no doubt be familiar: to propound a statement or series of statements and to ask the candidate to indicate which he accepts as true and which he rejects as false. The answer takes the form simply of letters or numbers, and the element of literary composition is completely absent. This retreat from the written word reaches its logical conclusion when the answers are reduced to the form of marks on a special answer sheet designed to be read at high speed by an electro-optical machine; the resulting digital information can then be passed to a computer for scoring and analysis.

The actual form in which the question is put has been the object of much experiment and inventiveness. In common with some other examiners, we feel that the proliferation of different types of question has become excessive and may, if all the available formats are combined in a single paper, lead to the testing of a candidate's mental agility rather than of his knowledge of the subject. However, a great deal of experience has now been accumulated with different formats, particularly in the United States, where they have been extensively used by the National Board of Medical Examiners and by many other organisations.

A full description of these formats was given by 1961 by

Hubbard and Clemans. Ten years later a further account by Hubbard (1971) made it clear that, in the light of experience, some of these formats had been found unsatisfactory and were no longer being used. There follows a brief review of some of the different types of MCQ which are or have been in use in the United States and in Britain. We have deliberately included some which have not stood the test of time as study of their shortcomings may be helpful in the design of new question formats.

American formats in current use

The simplest and most familiar format is the five-choice completion (the original one-from-five: Hubbard and Clemans Type a). This begins with a statement, or stem, followed by five 'completions'. The candidate is asked to choose which is the *best* completion to go with the stem. It should be noted that only one completion can be the right answer, also that, while some of the other completions may be definitely false, others may have an element of truth in them and are only 'wrong' in the sense that they are less satisfactory than the one 'best' answer.

Examples of this format follow:-
1. Tachycardia is best defined as
   A   an irregularity of heart rhythm
   B* an unusually rapid heart rate
   C   an unusually slow heart rate
   D   a left-to-right inversion of the usual cardiac anatomy
   E   an increase in heart rate occurring periodically with each inspiration

Here knowledge of a rather elementary sort is being tested; the correct definition of a technical term (in the CMP classification described in Chapter 2, (a) 'Knowledge of fundamental vocabulary ...'). The false items (the 'distractors') here are nearly all definable by other technical terms with which the student might confuse the subject of the question: C, bradycardia: D, dextrocardia: E, sinus arrhythmia.

2. Hodgkin's disease is an example of
   A   an autoimmune disease
   B   a nutritional disorder
   C   a virus infection
   D* a reticulosis
   E   a demyelinating disorder

Here again the knowledge is elementary and tests the candidate's understanding of categories (CMP (b) 'Understanding of concepts').

3. In the nephrotic syndrome, oedema is best explained by
   A   a rise in the osmotic pressure of the interstitial fluid
   B   a fall in the total osmotic pressure of the plasma
   C* a fall in the colloid osmotic pressure of the plasma
   D   a rise in the hydrostatic pressure in the capillaries
   E   an increase in capillary permeability to large molecules

This tests the candidate's knowledge of Starling's theory of the formation and reabsorption of tissue fluid, and his understanding of how this is disturbed in the formation of nephrotic oedema. There is only one right completion, C; the 'distractors' are all clearly wrong and no question of judgement arises. In terms of the CMP classification testing is mainly at the level of (b) 'Understanding of principles'.

4. A woman of 35 with known mitral incompetence complains of lassitude and night sweats. On examination, in addition to the cardiac murmur, a palpable spleen is found. The most important investigation would be
   A   determination of Brucella antibody titre
   B   determination of blood sedimentation rate
   C* blood culture
   D   examination of sputum for M. tuberculosis
  •E   splenic venography

Here the testing is in the area of CMP (c) 'Ability to understand and interpret data' and (d) 'Ability to solve relevant problems'. The candidate must first draw the conclusion that infective endocarditis is a possibility, and then select the most appropriate investigation for confirming this. An extension of this kind of management problem is described by Hubbard and Clemans as type g, and will be referred to later.

   This 'five-choice completion' is the most widely used MCQ format, and much experience has been gained from its use. However, it has one disadvantage which is sometimes serious: the difficulty of finding four plausible distractors. If, as one of the 'negatives', an absurdly unlikely choice is offered, it contributes little or nothing to the testing process and weakens the question. Generally little difficulty is found in devising two or perhaps three distractors; the fourth sometimes involves more work than the whole of the rest of the question put together.

   The next type of question to be considered is the 'five-choice association' (Hubbard and Clemans type b). A group of five entities is specified: then follows a list of other entities, each of which is related to one of the first group. For example:-

5.   A   Hyperparathyroidism
    B   Hyperthyroidism
    C   Hypothyroidism
    D   Diabetes mellitus
    E   Diabetes insipidus
    1. Delayed relaxation of tendon reflexes (C)
    2. Specific retinal changes (D)
    3. Increased phosphorus/creatinine clearance ratio (A)
    4. Low urine osmotic pressure with high plasma osmotic pressure (E)
    5. Tachycardia (B)
    6. Hoarse voice (C)
    7. Nephrotic syndrome (D)

On the whole this is not a versatile format and seems to test at a rather basic 'knowledge of facts' level.

A variation is the 'four-choice association' (type c) in which the relation is with one entity only, a second entity only, both entities or neither. Example:-

6. A   Aortic stenosis
   B   Aortic incompetence
   C   Both
   D   Neither
   1. Left ventricular hypertrophy (C)
   2. Opening snap (D)
   3. Anacrotic pulse (A)
   4. Diastolic murmur (B)

Again testing is at a rather basic factual level.

Another format described in Hubbard and Clemans' text (type g) is an application of the five-choice completion to the specific problems of clinical diagnosis and management. A case history is given together with a description of the findings on examination and the results of some simple investigations, and this material is made the basis for a sequence of five-choice questions, starting usually with the diagnosis and progressing to such problems as additional physical signs likely to be found, additional investigations desirable, treatment indicated and probable outcome.

A properly constructed problem of this type can place the candidate in just the situation of clinical uncertainty and of the need to choose the best option on the basis of incomplete evidence, with which every clinician is familiar. At the same time, patients do not present themselves bearing five-choice completion questions, and the chief drawback of this format as a realistic test of ability to manage a case is the way in which possible solutions (which the candidate might not have been able to think of unaided) are presented. Hubbard and Clemans' suggestion that the right diagnosis be omitted and replaced by an option, 'none of the above', seems to us a lame one in that there will still be no way of telling that the candidate has arrived at the right conclusion.

In type k (multiple completion) four numbered entities are listed and the candidate has to say what combination of these he would expect in the circumstances specified in the stem of the question. Example:-

7. The following are recognised manifestations of systemic lupus erythematosus:-
   1.   Nephrotic syndrome
   2.   Pericarditis
   3.   Raynaud's phenomenon
   4.   Recurrent renal stone formation
   A* 1,2 and 3 are correct
   B   1 and 3 are correct
   C   2 and 4 are correct
   D   Only 4 is correct

E 1, 2, 3 and 4 are all correct

The number of possible combinations of four options is 14, but in order to make the format compatible with an answer sheet allowing only five options, the possibilities are restricted as shown. A little investigation shows that the candidate can derive some useful hints from these restrictions. Thus, the solution (true or false) must *always* be the same for 1 and for 3. If 1 is false, 4 is always true. If 4 is false, 1 is always true. Suppose the candidate happens to know for certain that 1 is false; he can then deduce that 3 must be false and 4 true. The answer key then must be C or D and his uncertainty is reduced to whether statement 2 is true or false. This artificial restriction of the possibilities makes questions in this format both less effective and more tedious to construct, and we doubt whether they fully repay the trouble they cause to examiner and examinee alike. As we shall see, it is possible to pose this sort of question in a rather different format without any of the restrictions or 'built-in' information implicit in this type of question.

Discarded American formats

Type d ('excluded term'). This type of question is complicated and calls for detailed knowledge from the candidate (and a cool head in addition). The instructions read as follows:- 'There are two responses to be made to the following question. In the left-hand list are three lettered categories. Four of the five numbered items in the right-hand list are related in some way to *one* of these categories. Indicate (1) the letter of the category to which these four items belong, (2) the number of the item in the right-hand list which does *not* belong to the same category as the other four'. Example:-

8. A* Osteomalacia   1. Raised serum alkaline phosphatase
    B   Osteoporosis   2. Lowered serum phosphorus
    C   Osteitis fibrosa   3*. Bones painful only after fracture
                            4. Looser's zones in bone x-rays
                            5. Common in malabsorption syndrome

This format is without doubt too complicated, and has been the cause of much criticism of the MCQ technique in general.

Type e ('relationship analysis'). The candidate is confronted with two statements linked by the word 'because', and must select the correct relationship from the following:-
   A both statements true, second a correct explanation of the first
   B both statements true, second not a correct explanation of the first
   C first statement true, second false
   D first statement false, second true
   E both statements false

15

For example:-
9. In a facial paralysis of upper motor neurone type, the upper half of the face is spared BECAUSE the cortical neurones supplying the facial nucleus are never affected. (C)

This is a very effective format for testing the understanding of theory and of causal relationships, CMP classification (a) and (b). American examiners have evidently found it unsuitable for National Board examinations. We feel it may still have a place particularly in class tests where the teacher wishes to see how well he has conveyed to his students some theoretical concept.

Before turning to other formats, we may note an important point about those we have been considering. Most of them, and particularly the 'five-choice completion' (type a), require a single decision from the candidate rather than separate decisions about each completion. Thus, if the candidate recognises A as the best answer he is automatically rejecting B, C, D and E. When the question is asking what is the best management decision to take, this automatic rejection of the rest may be perfectly reasonable, if the distractors have been appropriately chosen. When the question deals with matters of factual recall, and the completions are not incompatible with one another, the fact that *only one* can be right may render the question less searching than it otherwise would be. This should be borne in mind when considering alternative formats.

The independent true-false format

Some examiners in Britain have found these American formats satisfactory; others have been concerned about their complexity. One outcome of a search for simpler formats has been the 'independent true-false' type which has been extensively used by several universities, notably Newcastle (where it originated), Birmingham, Liverpool and London, as well as by the Royal Colleges of Physicians, the Conjoint Board and other diploma-granting bodies. This type may bear a deceptive resemblance to the American type a, the five-choice completion, and if the two types are being used in the same paper very careful explanation to the candidates of the difference between them is needed. As with type a, the question begins with a stem, and is followed by a variable number of completions, any or all of which may be true or false. If, as is often the case, the number of completions is five, than the resemblance mentioned above becomes very marked. The composer of the question must take care not to include mutually incompatible completions and 'none of the above' can not be used. The format is in fact rather like the American type k (see p.14) but is a great improvement on it in that it is liberated from the strait-jacket of a choice of one combination out of five.

The 'independent true-false' is an extremely flexible and versatile format and it should be noted that the 'distractors' - completions to which the correct response is 'false' - require to be identified on their own merits rather than as less satisfactory answers than the single correct one in type a. This adds considerably to the power of the question. Thus each question requires as many decisions from the candidate as there are completions, compared with the single decision required for the type a question.

Some examples may illustrate this versatility. To begin with the most basic cognitive levels, we may test knowledge of terminology, CMP (a):-
10. The following are correct definitions or explanations:-
    A   Heberden's nodes: red, tender nodules in the palm or finger pulp in patients with infective endocarditis
    B* Ramsay Hunt syndrome: herpes zoster of the geniculate ganglion
    C   Pulsus alternans: an irregular pulse in which the beats occur in pairs, separated by a longer interval
    D   Osteomalacia: changes in the bone due to excessive secretion of parathyroid hormone
    E* Huntington's chorea: an inherited nervous disorder causing the development in middle life of choreiform movements and dementia

Here a deliberate attempt is made to explore possible areas of confusion; of the false statements, A describes Osler's nodes, C pulsus bigeminus and D osteitis fibrosa. Of the true statements, E requires a clear understanding of the difference between Huntington's chorea and Sydenham's chorea. No particular area of confusion arises with B, where all that is sought is accurate identification of the eponym of a rather uncommon condition.

Knowledge of specific facts, CMP (a) might be tested as follows:-
11. The following biochemical results are outside the accepted limits of normality:-
    A* Serum creatinine : 230μmol/l (2.5mg/100ml)
    B   Serum amylase : 120 Somogyi units
    C* Serum potassium : 6.5mmol/l (6.5mEq/l)
    D* Serum antistreptolysin O titre : 400 units/ml
    E   Serum uric acid (male patient) : 0.35 mmol/l (6 mg/100ml)

Moving to more complex areas, one might test knowledge and understanding of facts and concepts, CMP (a) and (b) by a question such as:-
12. Patients suffering from the nephrotic syndrome characteristically show
    A   a history of previous streptococcal infection
    B* heavy proteinuria
    C   a raised blood urea
    D* a lowered serum albumin
    E   a lowered serum globulin

To answer this correctly a candidate must have a clear idea of the concept of 'nephrotic syndrome' and of the mechanisms which operate to bring about the clinical phenomena.

Of particular importance in clinical medicine is the ability to understand and interpret data, CMP (c). Here we may test a candidate's ability to recognise significant points in a history:-

13. A man of 65 complains of pain in the back which came on abruptly three weeks ago following a violent fit of sneezing. He has also noticed lassitude and easy fatigue for three months. On examination he is pale; back movements are restricted and the lower lumbar spine is tender on percussion. The following diagnoses require serious consideration:-
    A   Osteoarthritis
    B*   Myelomatosis
    C   Paget's disease of bone
    D*   Secondary carcinoma
    E   Tuberculosis

Management problems, which may be classified under CMP (d) 'ability to solve relevant problems' and (e) 'judgement in evaluating a total situation' can also be effectively tested:-

14. A man of 40 with no previous history of illness has had three epileptic fits in the past 48 hours. There are no abnormal neurological signs. The following investigations are essential:-
    A*   Blood sugar
    B   Serum potassium
    C*   Serum test for syphilis
    D*   Chest X-ray
    E*   Serum calcium.

The construction of MCQs

Some suggestions about the technique of composing MCQs, and some examples of mistakes to be avoided, may be helpful at this point. These suggestions are framed in terms of the independent true-false format, with which we are most familiar, but the principles will be obvious and can be applied to most other formats.

Characteristics to be aimed at. 1. The stem and completions should be written in clear, unambiguous English. 2. Care should be taken to make *all* the completions follow on in a grammatical fashion from the stem. 3. Stem with completion should form a statement which is true or false in all circumstances without any room for argument. 4. Due thought should be given to the taxonomic level to be tested, the knowledge expected of the candidates and the importance of the subject-matter; in short, the objectives of assessment must be clearly defined.

Characteristics to be avoided. 1. There are certain indefinite words and expressions which are useful in everyday language but which make MCQs difficult or impossible to answer. Thus, characterisation of a statement as 'true' or 'false' may not be easy if it contains such words as 'usually', 'sometimes', 'rarely', 'often', 'occasionally'. Difficulties of this sort may well arise when questions about the clinical manifestations of disease are being composed. Some conventional expressions which have been found useful in this connection may be mentioned here; for example, a question might begin 'Recognised findings in ulcerative colitis include' and the completions could then be made up both of findings which were common or usual and also of those which were unusual but well recognised as associated, such as pyoderma gangrenosum. If the commoner findings only were being explored, the stem might be 'The following are characteristic of ulcerative colitis'. Narrowing the range still further, the candidate's knowledge of which features of the disease occur in all cases and which in only a proportion of the cases could be tested by a question beginning 'The diagnosis of ulcerative colitis should not be made in the absence of'.

2. Loose phrasing in which the distinction between random association and causal connection is lost should be avoided. The examiner may write 'The following may occur in ulcerative colitis' intending to find out whether the candidate knows which findings are part of the disease picture and which are not. However, for such a stem it is impossible to compose false completions which are logically sound. Obviously anything, from hallux valgus to Argyll-Robertson pupils, *may* occur in patients with ulcerative colitis; the question says nothing about causation. If the stem is rephrased to read 'Recognised manifestations of ulcerative colitis include' the ambiguity is removed.

3. The words 'always' and 'never' are probably best avoided. The occasions when they can be included in propositions about medical topics without any exceptions at all are few. Most candidates recognise this and regard their inclusion in a completion as an indication that the correct response is 'false'. The unwary may be caught out by a few propositions, usually depending on semantics or definitions, which admit of no argument; for example the statements 'in the nephrotic syndrome the urine always contains albumin' and 'in Addisonian pernicious anaemia the gastric juice never contains adequate amounts of intrinsic factor' are unequivocally true. However, such statements tend to be tautological and questions should not be designed to 'trick' the candidates.

Some examples of questions with faulty construction follow, together with suggestions for their improvement:-

15. The primary aims of treatment of respiratory failure are
    A   treatment of the primary cause
    B   adequate sedation

C   maintainance of airways
  D   artificial ventilation
  E   adequate antibiotic therapy

The faults here lie principally in the stem. 'Respiratory failure', without further definition, must include all cases of inadequate gas exchange in the lungs, and what would be a primary aim in one situation might well be of secondary importance in another. By the same reasoning the distinction between a 'primary' aim and all other aims must be largely artificial. This question was actually used in an examination in elementary medicine, the author's key being A, C. The first three completions caused little trouble but many candidates marked D and E as 'true', and indeed it would be hard to regard these as incorrect responses if the patient had respiratory paralysis (D) or pneumonia (E). On logical grounds one could also disagree with A and C as requiring a 'true' response in all cases. In some types of respiratory failure, for example in advanced emphysema or in mucoviscidosis, treatment of the cause may be impossible. In other types, for example in severe kyphoscoliosis, airways obstruction plays little part and is unlikely to require treatment. Completion B is a sound one which must be unequivocally false in all cases.

Useful modification of this question is difficult. Probably the best course would be to give up the attempt to establish completely general principles and instead to propose a specific example of respiratory failure, perhaps with a thumbnail clinical sketch:-

'A man of 65 with known long-standing chronic bronchitis and emphysema is admitted in severe respiratory distress. He is drowsy and cyanosed. His temperature is 38.5^0 C. Your management of this case would include'.

Specific measures could then be proposed and both sedation and the uncontrolled use of oxygen would make good negatives.

16. Oedema may be a clinical sign in
  A   chronic renal failure
  B   acute bronchitis
  C   liver failure
  D   hypertension
  E   acute circulatory failure (shock)

Here again the trouble lies in the stem; the distinction between association and causation is not made and as a result the only logical answer is 'true' to all five completions. The author's key was C and D but clearly in A heart failure could develop and so cause oedema. This presumably was the interpretation put upon A by 87 per cent of the candidates, who marked it as 'true'. In B and E some independent cause of oedema would have to be postulated and most candidates realised that this was not what was intended. Nevertheless 14 per cent and 28 per cent respectively marked these as 'true' and it seems likely that the confusion arose from the point under discussion rather than from a mistaken belief that acute bronchitis or circulatory failure could cause oedema per se.

A change of stem to 'Oedema is a recognised manifestation of' would be an improvement and B and E would then be firm negatives, though the status of D as a positive might then be contentious. Uncertainty would also arise from A, since hypertension is so common in renal failure. Perhaps a better (positive) completion would be 'nephrotic syndrome' or 'constrictive pericarditis'.

OTHER OBJECTIVE TECHNIQUES

As we have suggested above, the MCQ has certain compelling advantages which suggest that it will continue to play an important part in medical examinations in the foreseeable future. It also has disadvantages which make it undesirable as the *only* testing procedure, even in the cognitive domain. One drawback, which can be avoided if the examiners are sufficiently vigilant, is an insidious tendency to explore the 'small print' of medicine since rarities often lend themselves readily to the construction of MCQs. This is likely to have a bad effect on students approaching their final examination; if they know that questions in the past have dealt with such things as porphyria and thrombotic thrombocytopenic purpura they will spend time acquiring book-learning about these rarities, time which could be better spent learning more about commoner diseases or at the bedside. As we have said before, tests should be designed with clear-cut educational objectives in view.

Setting aside this objection, in the hope that it will be overcome by constant and critical scrutiny of the content of MCQs, we may turn to the consideration of those areas of cognitive testing for which the MCQ seems *not* to be the best solution. These are the areas in the CMP taxonomy of (d), (e) and (f) - analysis, evaluation and synthesis. In terms of clinical medicine such skills as pattern recognition, problem solving, diagnosis and the production of plans of investigation and management are involved. One disadvantage of the MCQ is that it imposes a certain rigidity on the framing of problems which in real life are often hedged about with 'ifs' and 'buts'. A more serious difficulty is inherent in the very structure of the MCQ: since the completions with which the candidate is confronted must include the right answer as well as some wrong ones, this may suffice to prompt his memory and help him to select the right one although, without this prompting, he might have been unable to recall it. This difficulty has been referred to above in connection with 'type g' questions and it takes its most acute form in just the area which this type is intended to cover, that of clinical diagnosis and management. If the simulation of clinical problems is to bear any sort of relation to real life, it seems essential that the candidate should make some response more spontaneous and positive than simply indicating a choice from five alternatives; in other words, we should ask the candidate to generate some response of his own, even if this amounts to no more than a single word.

If this point is conceded, it becomes clear that completely mechanical scoring of the responses is not possible. The examiner is once again, as in the case of essay questions, under the obligation to read the candidate's responses and to allot a score. However, it is possible for the scoring to be just as objective as with MCQs, if the acceptable answers have been agreed beforehand and allotted marks, according to their importance, on a pre-arranged scale (Fleming *et al.*, 1974). Team work is needed if large numbers of candidates are involved; for an entry of 500, 15 examiners can score 20 questions without difficulty in three to four hours.

This objective hand-marking system has been applied to three areas of testing: case-history problems, interpretation of laboratory data, and recognition of clinical and x-ray appearances in photographs. In the case-history problems, the candidate can be placed in the situation of a registrar dealing with a newly-admitted patient and his ability to make the necessary deductions from the clinical findings and to take the primary management decisions arising from these can be tested. The best material for testing at this level is the 'bread-and-butter' routine of ordinary clinical practice. Problems should be based on actual cases seen in the wards and in out-patient clinics. The histories should be presented in moderate detail. If, in an attempt to condense the history, all irrelevant and unimportant details are removed, the problem becomes unrealistic; if, on the other hand, all the detail is included it takes too long to read. Preliminary investigations such as blood-count and chest x-ray can be included but the problem is most suitable when the case is in an early stage of evolution and a wide range of possibilities still has to be considered. From the point of view of the examiner constructing the question this is often the best time at which to prepare the abstract and compose the questions. An example of this type of problem follows.

17. A 68 year old retired coal-miner was admitted because of an episode of unconsciousness 24 hours previously. While waiting at a railway station with his son he had fallen to the ground and was seen to move his arms and to roll his eyes; after about one minute he regained consciousness but then was unable to recognise his son. He had been somewhat confused since then. During the attack he was not incontinent of urine.
He had worked in a South Wales coal mine and at the age of 48 was told he had silicosis. He had had a cough with occasional sputum for many years. Of recent years he had noticed some shortness of breath on exertion but was not

seriously disabled. Otherwise his health had been good until the present episode.

He did not smoke. He drank 1 to 2 pints of Guinness per night and was not receiving any drugs.

During the previous two months his appetite had been poor and he thought he had lost about 6 Kg in weight. His wife had been away during this period visiting relatives.

On examination he did not appear markedly wasted. The blood pressure was 130/80 and the cardiovascular system was normal. The respiratory system was normal apart from crepitations at both lung bases. In the abdomen the liver was palpable 2 cm below the right costal margin; it was smooth and slightly tender. Examination of the nervous system showed that responses to questions and commands were very slow; his orientation in time and space was uncertain. Apart from nystagmus on looking to left and to right the cranial nerves appeared normal (testing of visual fields could not be done because of failure of co-operation). Power and tone in the limbs appeared normal; sensation could not be tested. There was a coarse tremor of both hands but co-ordination by the finger-nose test was normal. All tendon reflexes were present and symmetrical and the plantar responses were both flexor. The optic fundi showed minimal retinal arteriosclerosis. The urine contained no protein and no sugar and was normal on microscopy.

Four hours after admission he had a convulsion which began with movement of the arms and then passed through tonic and clonic phases. He was unconscious for three minutes in all. Immediately after the attack the right plantar response was extensor but the left remained flexor.

He continued in a state of mild confusion for the next two days. On the third day after admission his confusion became much worse, he became noisy and restless and appeared to be having visual hallucinations.

1. Give one immediate therapeutic action you would take.
2. What is the likeliest diagnosis?
3. Give three investigations which would be helpful in managing this case.

Questions on the interpretation of laboratory data also lend themselves well to this technique since the absence of the 'cueing' effect of MCQs is desirable here also. The clinical details can be much briefer and a question such as the following may be quoted as an example:-

18. A middle-aged man is admitted with severe shortness of breath. On examination he is drowsy and has moderate central cyanosis. Analysis of arterial blood yields the following results:-

PaO_2 6.9kPa   (52mmHg)
$PaCO_2$ 10.3kPa   (77mmHg)
pH   7.21

Actual bicarbonate 30.2mmol/l (30.2mEq/l)
1. What disturbance of acid-base equilibrium is present here?
2. Give two further investigations which would help you to plan treatment.

Pattern recognition may be tested in the same way by showing clinical photographs, x-rays, ECGs, photographs of gross morbid anatomical appearances or photomicrographs of histological sections. For example, a photograph of a boy of 12 with herpes zoster might be shown with these questions:-
19. 1. What is this rash?
    2. Give one reason why it might have occurred in this particular patient.

The need to avoid 'cueing' in such questions is obvious. However, by careful phrasing of questions, it is possible to use MCQs and at the same time to reduce 'cueing' to some degree. For example, questions for the photograph just mentioned might be as follows:-
20. The appearances in this photograph of a boy of 12 suggest
    A   a condition that is very common in this age-group
    B* a viral aetiology
    C   that severe itching was a prominent symptom
    D* that some disturbance of immunity was present
    E   that systemic treatment with idoxuridine would be beneficial

There is clearly room for experiment with MCQs along these lines but they are laborious to compose and more experience with their use is needed before they can be regarded as suitable for testing pattern recognition.

Another type of question requiring an answer of one or two words only may be called, for want of a better name, the 'missing link' (Fleming, 1975). Two terms, which may be symptoms, signs, diseases, syndromes or even drugs, are given and the candidate is required to provide a suitable link between them. If, for example the terms given were:-
21. Atrial fibrillation ...... fine tremor,
an acceptable link would be 'thyrotoxicosis'. Another example might be:-
22. Pulsus paradoxus ...... ascites,
for which 'constrictive pericarditis' would be a reasonable answer. Such questions seem not to have been very widely used as yet but, in our experience, they are capable of testing factual knowledge over a wide range and to any required depth. In addition they can be used as miniature clinical problem-solving exercises. Hand-marking is, of course, required and can be made objective by previous agreement on the acceptable

answers and on the scores to be allotted.

SHORT-ANSWER AND ESSAY QUESTIONS

Written verbal responses, restricted to a few words, a phrase, or at most a sentence, are evidently not far removed from the short-answer question, another well established testing technique. It is by no means unknown in traditional medical examinations, where it takes the form of 'Write short notes on ......'. Accurate specification of and agreement on what the answer must contain to be regarded as satisfactory is usually not difficult and it is possible to score questions of this sort in a fairly objective fashion. However, the answer will usually contain several sentences and the longer it is the greater the labour of scoring.

We must also consider the use, in present-day medical examinations, of the essay question. We have already touched on the arguments for rejecting this instrument in the testing of factual knowledge. Is there any place left for it in other areas of cognitive testing? We feel that it is still reasonable to use essay questions as an adjunct to other techniques, provided that they are designed so as to test attributes which cannot be tested satisfactorily otherwise and provided that the scoring process is preceded by thorough discussion between examiners. There must be agreement as to what attributes are being tested, what arguments or conclusions or solutions must be produced in order that the answer may be regarded as satisfactory, and what scores are to be allotted for these various points. Only in this way can any reasonable degree of objectivity and reliability of marking be obtained.

Those who favour the traditional essay claim that by its use it is possible to decide whether the candidate is capable of clear and logical reasoning and of original thought, and it is in this area that it seems likely to be most useful in cognitive testing. One possible basis for such an essay would be the case history problem discussed above, where the candidate could simply be asked to discuss the likely diagnosis, probable outcome including complications, and best lines of treatment, supporting his statements as far as possible with reasons. Or a question such as this might be used:-

23. Ten cases of serum hepatitis have occurred among the medical and nursing staff on two general medical wards of an 800-bedded district general hospital over a period of three months, the last case being diagnosed on Christmas Eve. Weekly returns of infectious diseases in Britain suggest that an epidemic of influenza is beginning. You have been asked to advise on the management of this situation. Describe the actions you would recommend, giving detailed reasons in each instance.

In our view, the more detail an essay question contains, the more likely it is to be effective in determining a candidate's capacity for logical reasoning.

PATIENT MANAGEMENT PROBLEMS

The testing of problem-solving ability has been approached in an original way by examiners in the U.S.A., who have developed the 'patient-management problem' (PMP). Here a clinical situation is presented, in much the same way as that considered above, but the possible management steps (investigation or treatment) are listed and the candidate makes his choice by removing, with a special eraser pencil, a layer of opaque plastic material over the area adjacent to the option offered. This reveals the consequences of his decision, e.g. the results of an investigation or the patient's response to therapy. One decision leads on to another and so through a stepwise chain of actions until (if these are correct) the patient recovers or responds favourably; if on the other hand the candidate has made a series of wrong decisions the patient becomes worse or may even succumb.

This format, the 'linear' version of the PMP, has been developed by the National Board of Medical Examiners (Hubbard, 1971). Experience with its use has shown that restriction to a single sequence of decisions leads to a somewhat artificial kind of problem and there is a tendency to move towards the 'branching' version as developed by McGuire and her associates at the University of Illinois (McGuire and Solomon, 1971). With this form it is possible to take account of the fact that different individuals may reach the same goal by a variety of paths and that there may not necessarily be a single correct path.

As is the case with many objective tests, some examiners find PMPs more difficult to construct than others. However, PMPs provide a useful and interesting means of discovering something of a candidate's capacities for problem-solving and decision-taking. There can be no doubt that they constitute a powerful and versatile testing technique although it is not free from the 'cueing' effect noted above in connection with MCQs. PMPs have not yet appeared on the British scene, because of the cost and complexity of producing the specially prepared answer sheets, the labour of devising the questions and the problems of scoring.

A still more sophisticated development involves transferring the whole problem to the data-store of a computer. The candidate communicates with the computer by means of a typewriter keyboard; the computer presents the problem in written form on a television screen and records the results of the candidate's responses. A startling impression of a real clinical encounter can be created, though the answers provided by the computer may be more logical than those obtained from actual patients, despite the pains taken by those in charge of the construction of such test programs to use the patient's own words as far as possible. Psychomotor interviewing skills, such as a candidate's ability to appreciate that the difficulty he is having in getting any coherent response from his patient is due to dementia, mental retardation or the influence of drugs, need, of course, to be tested in some other way.

Much time is being devoted to the refinement of the computer-based examination in North America. Some centres use an 'index' approach (in which only a limited, though extensive, number of areas of enquiry are available) and others the 'free language' approach which allows much wider scope to the candidate, though it involves a more complex computer program and provides greater difficulties in scoring.

These techniques call for large managerial and secretarial resources. If ever a centralised medical examinations service is set up in Britain, test procedures such as these might be within its grasp. Examining authorities such as universities, colleges and specialty boards are unlikely to dispose of the resources required.

Problem-simulation of this sort is evidently not a practical proposition in Britain at present as a test procedure. However, as a teaching method it must command serious attention. The computer simulation in particular recalls the instruction devices developed by aircraft companies for training pilots to fly new types of aircraft without leaving the ground. In the same way, doctors in training can be given the experience they need by being placed in difficult clinical situations without any fear of harm being done to an actual patient.

Other presentations of test material by audio-visual techniques are possible. We have already commented on the use of projected slides and x-ray films; the same idea can be extended to involve the use of recorded heart sounds and breath sounds, cine-film or video-tape recordings of dynamic phenomena such as pulsation of neck veins, delayed relaxation of tendon reflexes or abnormal gaits, and video-tape recordings of interviews between doctors and patient (this last having special application to testing in psychiatry).

ORAL EXAMINATIONS

Finally we must consider the place of the oral examination in cognitive testing. As we have said, in the age of innocence in medical examinations this was the only test instrument. However, use of the oral is seriously hampered by the limited area of knowledge that can be explored in the time available and by its notorious unreliability, due to variable marking standards and to arbitrary selection of subjects by examiners. Now that techniques so much better suited to testing in the cognitive domain have been developed, we think it may fairly be said that *in this field* the oral has been completely superseded and that a case can be made for confining its use to testing in the affective domain, where it may have advantages.

REFERENCES

Dudley, H.A.F. (1973) Multiple-choice tests: time for a second look? *Lancet, 2*, 195.

Fleming, P.R. (1975) M.L.Q. : A Supplement to M.C.Q. *Lancet, 2,* 601.

Fleming, P.R., Manderson, W.G., Matthews, M.B., Sanderson, P.H. and Stokes, J.F. (1974) Evolution of an Examination: M.R.C.P. (U.K.). *British Medical Journal,* 1,99.

Hubbard, J.P. (1971). *Measuring Medical Education.* Philadelphia: Lea and Febiger.

Hubbard, J.P. and Clemans, W.V. (1961) *Multiple-choice Examinations in Medicine.* Philadelphia : Lea and Febiger.

McGuire, C. and Solomon, L. (1971) *Clinical Simulations: Selected Problems in Patient Management.* New York: Appleton-Century-Crofts.

4. Psychomotor Skills

Though the idea of psychomotor skills is equated in many people's minds with a clinical examination involving a human patient, these skills are in fact also assessed in the earlier phases of a medical student's training, usually leaving a lasting impression on his mind.

Few doctors are without a memory of the choking horror following an over-confident incision into the ventral surface of an earthworm only to find that the whole of its dorsal neural apparatus had been destroyed; or of the despairing discard of a supersaturated solution at the end of a three hour pharmacology practical into the cold water sink from which splendid crystals could be rescued by the hasty insertion of the plug just in time to determine their melting point; or of the frustration of the Gram stain that imparted a neutral tint, neither red nor purple, to the bacterium which was hopefully labelled as a diphtheroid in the blind conviction that the examiner could not possibly have wished to expose candidates to a pathogenic organism.

We have already accepted that the do-it-yourself approach to such bench experiments is a valuable aid to understanding, but it is questionable whether a formal examination of such techniques is likely to yield meaningful results. This is an area in which it seems to us that continuous assessment could be most usefully applied, and, indeed, many universities already evaluate psychomotor skills of this kind by ensuring that a candidate has carried out a sufficient number of practical experiments or dissections in the course of his training. The pattern over the country as a whole is uneven, and we must reiterate our belief that it is at this stage more logical to test the extent to which knowledge and understanding have been acquired rather than the method of their acquisition. Doctors will not need to demonstrate the mouth-parts of a cockroach during their practising career.

THE CLINICAL EXAMINATION

The British have no special reputation as distinguished dissectors of dogfish or as unerring exposers of the spheno-palatine ganglion, but we do set great store by our expertise at the bedside, the evaluation of which must now be examined in more detail. Clinical method is also valued in developing countries which recognise that, though they have pressing problems to solve in the epidemiological field, these can be approached only from a firm base of reliable data-gathering which demands something more than a purely demographic training. And in the USA there is a resurgence of interest in psychomotor skills which may have been undervalued for a while as a result of the necessary emphasis laid on basic science and technology by the Flexner report (Flexner, 1910).

In Britain, the 'clinical' has survived as the keystone of examinations at graduate and postgraduate level in medicine, surgery, obstetrics and gynaecology and paediatrics. Candidates know that they cannot pass the examination as a whole unless they pass its clinical component.

The candidate usually spends up to an hour with a single 'long case' at the end of which time he is expected to discuss the history and physical signs with two examiners working together for fifteen to twenty minutes.

He is then asked to examine specific aspects of the clinical state in other patients, ('report on the cardiac state of this man who is short of breath', 'examine the legs of this patient who has difficulty in walking') and discuss his findings with two other examiners for a similar period.

One of the serious weaknesses of the 'clinical' is immediately apparent, namely the assessment of the candidates' skill in dealing with only one type of patient in the 'long case'. The luck of the draw plays too dominant a part in determining the examiners' judgement; a candidate may perform well if faced by a respiratory problem but find himself all at sea in neurological territory; the reliability of this part of the examination must be suspect.

If examiners' enquiries were confined to symptoms and signs and their interpretation, improvement might be expected, but this is often not so. It is probably a combination of these two weaknesses that have led cynics to regard the 'clinical' as the sacred cow of British medicine and its harsher contemporary critics to categorise it as a half-hour disaster session.

Criticisms of the clinical examination

It is certainly surprising that the 'clinical' has come in for so little comment during an era in which essay papers and oral confrontations have been so severely challenged. This may well be the result of examiners instinctively recognising that this part of the examination provides them with the best chance of preserving the traditional professional species by making appropriate 'phenotype' judgements, and it is certainly true that the 'clinical' has been used for different purposes by different examiners at different times over the years, not simply for the assessment of psychomotor skills. This is the main reason why its performance has been found to be uneven when it has been scrutinised. Examiners take account, in varying proportion, of the candidate's capacity to

(a) extract a relevant history (including social and family background),
(b) seek and elicit abnormal physical signs,
(c) synthesise this information into a differential diagnosis,
(d) devise a reasonable framework of investigation,
(e) reach a firm diagnosis,
(f) treat,
(g) give a prognosis,
(h) convey the gist of his conclusions to the patient and his family.

In addition, they may take account of whether the candidate is clean, gentle, assured or over-confident, talkative or taciturn, whether his hands are more often in his pockets than on the patient's pulse, whether his tie indicates membership of an acceptable club and, in the case of a female, whether she is neatly or ostentatiously clad. Some completely fail to control the atavistic feelings which come to the surface when confronted with a woman at their mercy; others act out deep-seated Galahad complexes of which they remain blissfully unaware (Stokes, 1967).

The patient in the clinical examination

It is clear that examiners in the 'clinical' have been given insufficient guidance as to what is expected of them, but there is also a need to look more closely at the type of patient who is pressed into service for the examination. Too often these have been 'professionals' who have made themselves easily available to hard-pressed registrars entrusted with the organisation of the examination. Considering the central role they play, their financial remuneration is, in general, paltry, so they cannot do it for the money; it is probably the power which attracts them, the opportunity to suppress a vital piece of history, occlude a physical sign and so influence a candidate's chance of passing; this may occur at a subconscious level and the most chronic professional patients like to constitute themselves as assistant examiners in which role some of them have become quite skilled.

Examiners have recognised this behaviour and have, partly for this reason, made a point of being present at the bedside with the candidate during his examination of the 'short case' at which the ability to collect physical signs is tested. But time does not usually permit him to observe the candidate at work on the history; this may be one reason why the 'long case' has not functioned well in the past, the history receiving insufficient scrutiny or emphasis (though history-taking is probably the most important element in clinical practice). The confrontation between examiner and examinee often degenerates into a theoretical discussion of the relative merits of the various serological tests for syphilis after the Argyll Robertson pupils and the Charcot's joints have led to a confident diagnosis of tabes dorsalis in the first five minutes.

'Short cases' have, on the whole, served their purpose better in the past, though there has been a danger of including rare constellations of signs, representing a disease which is either recognised at once or not at all and which may never be encountered again in an individual's professional lifetime; this danger exists particularly in paediatrics with its wide range of FLK (Funny Looking Kids) syndromes, but it is present in adult medicine too. It must be emphasised that short cases should not constitute a series of 'spot' diagnoses but should be used to test a candidate's skill in clinical method over as wide a range as time permits.

IMPROVEMENT IN RELIABILITY BY THE USE OF SIMULATION TECHNIQUES

The evident unreliability of the traditional clinical examination as a result of the factors outlined and the well-known and inevitable difference in judgements between different examiners and in varying circumstances of the same examiner have led to much effort in North America to synthesise tests of clinical competence from which the variable of the patient and the variable of the examiner have been excluded, leaving the variable of the candidate for assessment.

These tests, such as the patient-management problems, do not lie in the psychomotor domain and cannot, therefore, be completely satisfactory substitutes for the clinical examination; rather, they form a part of the problem-solving and decision-making components of the cognitive domain and, as such, are discussed in Chapter 3.

Use of models in place of the patient

Denson and Abrahamson's (1969) development of Sim I, a monumental piece of bio-engineering, has provided an opportunity of testing the psychomotor skills of the anaesthetist by automatically scoring the consequences of his actions as he passes an endotracheal tube down the model's throat, and observes in the model's pupils what happens when he injects a drug into the model's antecubital vein. Sim I is a useful training device in a limited field and it does not need much imagination to see how its central ingenious idea might be applied to other parts of the body, with interchangeable tapes of recorded heart sounds inserted into a model thorax and a variety of organs, the seat of disease, put into a model abdomen to be explored either by palpation or by pelvic examination. Doubtless the technical problems could be overcome, but the cost at present is prohibitive. Sim I remains, however, a pioneering example of how the elicitation of at least some physical signs might possibly be tested in an objective way without the help of a patient who would become exhausted if exposed to many candidates.

Nevertheless, however realistic a model might be, we have an intuitive preference for the use of live patients in a clinical examination.

Use of trained non-patients in place of the patient

Most human beings, whether they are examiners, faculty staff, professional actors or city housewives, are capable of simulating a patient up to a point if they are given enough skilled coaching and rehearsal. The simulation for the most part must be confined to giving a history, but Barrows (1971) at McMaster University has extended the concept of a simulated patient to include physical signs in the neurological area. His Hamilton housewives are able to produce exaggerated tendon reflexes, cogwheel rigidity and extensor plantar responses as well as sensory deficit at will and in this restricted area it may be possible to provide all the clinical data that a candidate might be expected to assemble as a result of contact with a real patient.

A candidate's capacity to handle an awkward situation may also be tested by confronting him with a trained 'patient' playing the part of the mother of a child who has just been discovered to have leukaemia, or of a middle-aged labourer on the bread-line whose unexplained back pain demands hospital investigation.

CONTINUOUS ASSESSMENT OF CLINICAL COMPETENCE

No-one would deny that an ability to take a history and discover abnormal physical signs is an important part of a doctor's competence, though, in common with many others, we doubt whether its formal testing is best carried out at a *graduating* examination. The claim can fairly be made that 'I give my students a clinical examination on every ward round' and it is unreasonable to suggest that two pairs of examiners are able to take a more meaningful decision on the basis of a candidate's handling of two patients than the teachers under whose guidance he has been learning for several years. The case for serial assessment of the undergraduate during his training is a strong one; it does demand, however, that there is a faculty policy and some agreement on the standards required, that a check list of clinical capabilities is drawn up, that special responsibility for a group of students is vested in one member of the staff, that there are enough staff to go round, that careful records of all students are kept and that some arrangement is made, possibly by the use of external examiners, to ensure that standards of performance do not diverge too widely between one school and another. All this puts a considerable strain on the Dean's office, which is less well supported in Britain than in North America, and on the medical school staff who are numerically less strong.

Nevertheless it is a reasonable aim which will be discussed further in Chapter 9.

THE NEED FOR A FORMAL CLINICAL EXAMINATION

Undergraduate level

If it is felt that it is necessary to hold, in addition, a formal 'clinical' at the end of undergraduate training, either to ensure comparable standards with other schools or to provide evidence for the student that clinical skills are still considered important, then there is much to be said for a single integrated 'clinical' at which the candidate's response to any kind of patient may be judged. The technique of history-taking does not vary as between a medical, surgical or obstetrical case and it is not difficult to observe whether a student has been in the habit of examining a patient whatever the nature of the patient's problem. Many medical cases become surgical and vice versa. The possible exception lies in paediatrics where special skills of physical examination may be needed and the history is usually taken through a third person. Psychiatric history-taking, too, may prove awkward to test, and discussion of videotaped interviews between psychiatrist and patient may have a part to play here.

Postgraduate level

It is at the postgraduate level in Britain that the need for a formal 'clinical' remains. This is due to the fact that our postgraduate training programmes are as yet rudimentary and we are not in a position to rely wholly on the judgement of those clinicians under whom postgraduates are training. With limited opportunities for specialist training it is also necessary to have some sort of gate through which a candidate might be asked to pass on his way to further training. This need is sharpened by the large numbers of doctors from overseas who continue to seek postgraduate training in Britain and who are looking for some yardstick by which to measure their performance. Though it may be possible to sort these men out in their homelands up to a point by such examinations as the Primary FRCS and the Common Part I MRCP (UK) overseas, the clinical capabilities of those postgraduates who are selected for training in Britain remain variable. So long as the countries who sponsor them expect them to return home with a British diploma, the need for a 'clinical', the hallmark of British medicine, remains. There is, of course, a danger here; ideally, developing countries should devise their own postgraduate diplomas and give them due weight when selecting men for career posts in government medical service; only in this way can they ensure a supply of doctors who have learned the skills which are needed for subsequent work in the areas in which their domestic problems lie.

THE DESIGN OF THE CLINICAL EXAMINATION

In the meantime we are obliged to make our 'clinical' as fair and reasonable a test as possible. It suffers at present from the two common shortcomings of so many examinations, namely limited range and examiner variability.

Short cases

Extended coverage can be made in the 'short case' section, if it is understood and accepted that it is only, for instance, necessary for a candidate to demonstrate that he can feel for and find enlarged lymph nodes in the neck, rather than show, in addition, a knowledge of the histopathology of Hodgkin's disease and the niceties of its treatment; that it is enough for him to make a direct move to test the pupillary reaction after he has observed unilateral ptosis rather than rehearse the differential diagnosis of Horner's syndrome. It should be possible to test a candidate's psychomotor skill in physical examination in four or five separate systems in twenty minutes. Some types of case clearly take longer than others, cardiac or pulmonary for instance, and it is in these that virtue may be found in a check list of things which need testing. In the cardiovascular system, the examiner might be asked to make a definitive judgement on a five-point scale on a candidate's capacity (a) to report on the apex beat; (b) to comment meaningfully on the jugular venous pulse; (c) to decide what valvular lesions or rhythm abnormalities are present. Such structuring of a 'short case' test can be tedious and sometimes irritating to examiners but it can be expected to improve the reliability of the assessment and has been shown to do so by Harden *et al.* (1975). Part of the reluctance to accept such a manoeuvre doubtless stems from the fact that a clinical confrontation provides examiners with an opportunity of making a judgement on and giving weight to such qualities as poise, likeability and capacity for making good rapport with a patient. There is no doubt at all that these attributes are important in determining the effectiveness of a doctor's work, and any move towards structuring a clinical examination must acknowledge this and ask for separate evaluation by the examiner in this nebulous but crucial area which is in danger of becoming undervalued since it has rarely, so far, been formally assessed. This problem is considered further in Chapter 5.

Long case

The 'long case' with whom the candidate spends more time, should be the subject of more detailed enquiry, particularly as to history-taking, which remains one of the most important medical exercises and one of the more difficult to test. Patients who take part in the examination as 'long cases' should be patients who are in hospital with a live problem; they need not show any abnormal physical signs but should have the full and sometimes complex history that is found in, say, ulcerative colitis, ischaemic heart disease, asthma, diabetes, peptic ulceration, depression and hypertension. Their total case records should be available to the examiners. Ideally, the timing of the traditional 'clinical' should be arranged so as to allow an examiner to sit in with the candidate for at least part of the time he is taking the history in the same way as the examiner now commonly, and rightly, spends time at the bedside with the candidate while he is eliciting his physical signs. This does not occur now and this omission is one of the weak points of the 'long case'.

In addition to assessing history-taking, the examiner can, at this point, make a judgement on the total summing-up of the case by the candidate and on his capacity for making a management plan to meet the situation. A separate evaluation of the candidate's general attributes, referred to above, can be made at the same time - by a different examiner.

Briefing the examiner

The need for briefing examiners and for pre-test meetings to ensure that everyone knows what he is supposed to be doing cannot be over-emphasised. This is specially true if check lists are used, but at any clinical examination part of the unreliability derives from uncertainty in the examiner's mind as to what criteria and standards should be applied.

Even in the absence of formal training courses for examiners, a great deal can be achieved by group discussions and mutual clarification of ideas before the 'clinical' starts. Unless briefing discussions take place, individual examiners may forget that the purpose of the 'clinical' should be to test clinical method and will be in danger of using valuable bedside time in straying into the area of factual recall, which is better tested in other sections of the examination.

Variability of examiners

However much trouble is taken in securing agreement among examiners before the 'clinical' on exactly what it is that they are going to look for and how they are going to score it, the difficulties of the variability of examiners' judgement still remain. An expression of deep dismay may be seen to settle on a candidate's face when he finds himself confronted by a notorious hawk, in contrast to the glow of relief (sometimes misplaced) engendered by a celebrated dove. It is possible, if careful records are kept of individual examiners' judgements over several examinations to analyse them and construct a hawk/dove rank order, releasing to an individual examiner at his request, his position on the 'ladder', though it would not be desirable to provide any further details. For such a rank order to be meaningful, it is, of course, essential for each individual examiner to write down his own score separately before consultation with his colleagues and before any verbal or facial signals have been exchanged; otherwise analysis tends to show no more than who is the dominant examiner of a pair or of a group who meet to agree a final score of the candidate's performance in the clinical section of the examination. It is now generally agreed that examiners should not work singly, that is that no candidate should be confronted by a solitary examiner; one examiner should interrogate, the other listen, both assess. At the end of the confrontation with the candidate each examiner should write down his own independent score; a final score should then be agreed after discussion (Stokes, 1974).

The effort involved in designing a clinical examination along these lines, including the logistical planning, which is discussed in Chapter 8, is considerable. Nevertheless it will be adequately rewarded if the candidates feel that they have had a squarer deal than has sometimes been the case in the past and if examiners, by discussing freely the issues involved before the examination takes place, feel that their heavy responsibilities are easier to discharge.

TESTING MORE COMPLEX SKILLS

It is evident that we have only scratched the surface of the evaluation of psychomotor skills. As we have remarked, the clinical examination tends to be erected around what material is readily available and comparatively easy to organise; it can only take us a certain distance.

Surgical evaluation in the past has sometimes included the dissection of a cadaver but even this did not give very satisfactory evidence of what a man could do with a living body. Examinations in obstetrics and gynaecology do not tell us whether a candidate is capable of applying forceps in a non-traumatic way or of dealing with obstructed labour. In medicine there is no formal test of a man's capacity to perform a lumbar puncture or a paracentesis, or even to pass a urethral catheter or to enter a vein. Quite apart from the difficulties of arrangement, ethical considerations demand that these skills be learned under supervision in the course of training. Perhaps they should be more formally tested during this training. It would imply too rigid an approach to demand that a postgraduate should be 'signed up' for ten appendicectomies, but we should recognise that there is a problem. It might be that some form of check list should be used; this would be particularly needed if a specialist register were introduced in the future, so that it would be possible to make a statement at the end of a man's training in gastroenterology, for example, that he was known to be capable of doing a liver biopsy and of performing an endoscopy.

REFERENCES

Barrows, H.S. (1971) *Simulated Patients*. Springfield, Illinois: Charles C. Thomas.
Denson, J.S. and Abrahamson, S. (1969) A Computer-Controlled Patient Simulator. *Journal of the American Medical Association*. 208, 504.
Flexner, A. (1910). *Medical Education in the United States and Canada*. Boston; The Merrymount Press.
Harden, R. McG., Stevenson, M., Downie, W.W.W. and Wilson, G.M. (1975). Assessment of Clinical Competence Using Objective Structured Examination. *British Medical Journal* 1, 447.
Stokes, J.F. (1967) Examining in the United States : The National Board of Medical Examiners. *British Journal of Medical Education* 1, 320.
Stokes, J.F. (1974) *The Clinical Examination*. Medical Education Booklet No.2. Dundee. Association For The Study Of Medical Education.

5. Assessment of Professional Attitudes

An attitude is a frame of mind, a feeling for or against something. All doctors have attitudes which are relevant to their work; they hold attitudes as medical teachers, for example, about the importance of assessing attitudes.

Attitudes can be defined with some degree of precision and are conventionally classified in the 'affective domain', that is the component of mental performance concerned with feeling and emotion. We have detailed in Chapter 2 the qualities desirable in a doctor as set out by Charvat, McGuire and Parsons (1968). Consideration of such qualities as 'recognition of medical capabilities and limitations' and 'ability to establish effective relationships with colleagues' makes it clear that an attitude is not simply a matter of feeling. Combined with the emotion is included, in addition, a cognitive element (knowledge) and also a tendency to action. Thus, in the simplest possible terms, without knowledge there can be no feeling, and feeling itself is likely to be followed by action. For example, a clinical teacher faced by a proposal to increase the emphasis on behavioural sciences in the teaching of his own subject may react as follows. Basing his judgement on his own knowledge, such as it is, of psychology he may become impatient or even angry when any extension in the teaching of psychology into his own subject is discussed; in all probability he will translate this attitude into action or at least argument at a meeting of a curriculum committee. It is not difficult to recognise similar trains of mental events when doctors express attitudes towards any emotionally-charged or debatable topic such as abortion, the treatment of spina bifida, the management of suicide attempts, or the fluoridation of water.

All attitudes are learned. The attitudes which medical students bring with them to medical school become modified and supplemented during the course of their training in ways which may or may not be desirable; these attitudes can be inferred from the student's behaviour. Favourable attitudes are 'approach tendencies', negative attitudes 'avoidance tendencies'. For example, a student interested in psychiatry will react to his psychiatric instruction quite differently from the student with a negative attitude to psychiatry; this has clear implications for the different teaching methods needed for these two students.

Because professional attitudes are inferred from actual behaviour, the teacher must specify the kind of behaviour which will be taken to indicate a particular attitude. If a student misses many sessions of teaching about a subject such as ophthalmology the teacher can infer from his non-attendance that he is probably not interested in that specialty. The tendency of students to vote with their feet is well-known.

CAN ATTITUDES BE EXAMINED ?

Professional attitudes can be assessed. Teachers regularly pay attention to the professional attitudes of students and quite informally make judgements based on what they see a student do. Thus, if he acts so as to appear to his teacher as responsible, considerate to patients and colleagues, active in tutorials and at the bedside and increasingly knowledgeable, the teacher will react favourably. If a student, by contrast, is idle, inattentive, inactive and perfunctory about his obligations to colleagues and to patients, the teacher will take an adverse view of his performance.

Despite this, formal assessment of attitudes still plays little or no part in professional examinations. The most likely reason for this neglect is that medical examiners may be reluctant to penalise candidates on the basis of their *subjective* opinions, being instinctively aware that such opinions are open to all the errors of intuitive judgements. These errors can be greatly reduced by paying attention to two requirements. The first is to define accurately and in detail the professional attitudes to be assessed. The second is to be sufficiently familiar with the principles of attitude measurement to be able to record judgements in a reliable form. Lack of attention to these points is conspicuous in the traditional assessment of attitudes by examiners. For example, if, in a clinical examination, a candidate palpates a patient's abdomen roughly or with cold hands and the patient winces, the examiner is likely to be unfavourably impressed. A candidate who is offhand, inattentive and curt in an oral examination is also liable to be marked down. This informal approach is inadequate because (a) not all candiates are being tested for the warmth of their palms prior to abdominal palpation and therefore this part of the test is not standarised and (b) even for the occasional candidate who, on a chance basis, is subjected to this test, the extent of the penalty is not laid down but depends on the fluctuating and subjective judgement of the examiner. Thus, neither the requirement for precise definition nor that for reliable measurement has been met.

In order to improve the reliability of this assessment, examiners may be provided with a list of attributes and given a scale of ratings according to which the candidates are to be evaluated. A rating is an estimate, made according to some systematised procedure, of the degree to which a person possesses a given characteristic, and may be expressed qualitatively or quantitatively. For example, in a postgraduate clinical

examination in psychiatry, the examiners may be asked, after observing each candidate examine his patients and hearing his subsequent report on them, to rate him according to a scale: 1 (superior); 2 (satisfactory); 3 (unsatisfactory), on the following attributes:-
    (a)   Appropriateness of understanding about the clinical phenomena elicited
    (b)   Rapport with patient
    (c)   Judgement exercised
    (d)   General treatment ability
    (e)   Psychotherapeutic ability
    (f)   Estimate of personal stability of trainee.

It will be evident that many examiners will be hesitant to commit themselves after a single observation about item (e), and still more will object to inclusion of item (f), with good reason declining to make so complex a judgement at one point in time, when in any case special stresses operate.

    Continuous assessment by tutors in the course of a student's or doctor's training provides an important contribution to evaluation in this area. The American Board of Orthopaedic Surgery do not ask their examiners to rate professional attitudes at the time of the examination. Instead, a Candidate Evaluation Form (Levine and McGuire, 1971) is sent to four orthopaedic surgeons who have personal knowledge of the candidate, and they rate him on 10 factors, which include relationships with patients and with colleagues, continuing responsibility and moral and ethical values.

    To assist the teachers in completing the form, each factor is illustrated by a list of positive and negative actions relating to that factor. Candidates are rated on a 12-point scale from Poor to Excellent. The ratings for each candidate are averaged and weighted by the Board. The resulting profiles are then reviewed by the Committee on Eligibility which decides whether applicants may take the examination.

    The first item in the Evaluation Form is the professional attitude of establishing adequate relationships with patients. A doctor is expected to be able to obtain co-operation from patients, to relieve their anxiety and to instil confidence. At the same time he is expected to stand back and not become too emotionally involved. 'Detached concern' is a term often applied to this set of attitudes. He is expected to convey to the patient that any problem may be confided to him, and that he will not be judgemental and certainly not censorious.

    The second quality required of the future orthopaedic surgeons, clinical responsibility, denotes the trainee's willingness to accept the responsibility for long-term patient care. This is an attribute which it is difficult to judge at one point in time and which becomes particularly important after graduation, during the later phases of medical training and in actual practice. A main component in clinical responsibility is dependability; a person showing this is consistent and can be counted on to fulfil expectations; he makes commitments and carries them through. A second component is initiative; the person does more than the situation requires, exercising foresight in anticipating difficulties and their solution, and showing a thoroughness which goes beyond what is expected. A third component of clinical responsibility is altruism in that benefit to others is a major consideration in the student's actions.

Dependability, initiative and altruism may be descriptions of behaviour too abstract for an examiner to observe and rate. He needs clearer criteria by which to judge clinical responsibility. Evidence of responsibility may be shown by such behaviour as: (a) sensitivity to the needs and feelings of patients, (b) effective decision-making, (c) treating others to the best of one's ability and in a way one would wish to be treated oneself, (d) meeting obligations, (e) responding to perceived needs of others, and (f) accountability - being answerable for one's actions both to oneself and to others.

Each of these aspects of behaviour can then be presented on a graphic rating scale, i.e. a continuous straight line with cues or categories along the line to guide the rater. For example:- 'Is this candidate responsive to the needs and feelings of patients ?'

Extremely   Usually   Only occasionally   Hardly   Not at all

By specifying the factors to be rated in such operational detail, the reliability of ratings can be increased sufficiently to justify their use in examinations (Levine and McGuire, 1971).

SHOULD ATTITUDES BE ASSESSED IN PROFESSIONAL EXAMINATIONS ?

There is still disagreement within the medical profession as to whether attitudes should be given weight in examinations. Reitsma (1973) quoted a troubled medical school teacher at Utrecht who had to rate a student's performance after a clinical clerkship in paediatrics. 'This student gave the correct answers to the searching questions I asked him. He was skilful and knew his job. I thought of giving him a mark of 8, but he had not been good in the wards. He went about in a rather arbitrary way with criticism about everybody and everything, and got everybody's back up. So I gave him only a mark of 6. A colleague of mine claimed, however, that I should have given him the higher mark, as his behaviour had nothing to do with it. Should I have awarded the higher or the lower mark ?'

We believe that professional attitudes are of great importance and highly relevant not only to the career advice given to students and young doctors, but also to subsequent performance in professional practice. We also believe that they should be assessed more formally than hitherto. However, such an assessment demands, as in all other aspects of evaluation, a clear definition of objectives in terms of desirable attributes and behaviour. For example, the Dutch student could claim, perhaps justifiably, that his paediatrics attachment did not set out to train him in team skills or good personal relationships.

MEASURING ATTITUDES

If it is accepted, as we believe it should be, that attitudes can only be reliably assessed in the course of training, it becomes possible to make use of such assessments in two distinct ways. They may, and should, play some part in the final assessment of a candidate at the end of a course of training (*summative* evaluation). Even more important is their role in systematic evaluation throughout a course of instruction. Here they have a homeostatic monitoring function, providing the student with a constant flow of feed-back as he moves from one phase of training to another. Corrective actions can be taken by both student and teacher long before misconceptions become ingrained and failure inevitable. In such a system the attitudinal assessment is part of the *formative* evaluation.

When attitudes are evaluated, the necessary observations may be provided either by teachers who judge the students, or the observations may be elicited directly from students. We have already noted the ways in which teachers may contribute to such judgements. Measures which call on students to provide information by completing forms consist either of questionnaires or, more elaborately, of rating scales. The procedures for devising questionnaires are well-documented but are often not followed; perfunctory questionnaires, as Flexner (1930) noted, result in 'information or non-information, one never knows which'.

Questionnaires

A number of step-like preparations are involved in the development of a questionnaire. The investigator has to make a decision about the kind of information required, and the best questions for obtaining such information. A most important consideration is whether the questionnaire will be administered verbally by an interview, or whether it will be of postal type. A necessary step is to decide in advance how the information obtained will be used, and how the responses will be analysed; all 'interesting' issues, which are not relevant and useful, should be firmly excluded.

The investigator must understand the subject he plans to study. Much misinformation results from questionnaires constructed by investigators unfamiliar with medical education and medical students. Often, preliminary study of the students must precede the wording of questionnaire items. This study may take the form of group discussions or individual interviews with students; pilot surveys will also be called for to develop the items, and to frame questions in appropriate language which is unambiguous. In phrasing questions, potential bias likely in the responses must be anticipated. The investigator needs to avoid putting words into his subjects' mouths. When one asks a respondent if he agrees or disagrees with a proposition, the subject of the proposition is put into his mind. Open-ended questions reveal whether a subject is already in the respondent's mind. It is necessary to avoid leading questions, excessively abstract questions, irritating questions, demanding questions which are long and complicated and generalised and hypothetical questions (e.g. 'How would you rate the opportunity for satisfying medical practice in the United Kingdom?'). All these erroneous forms of words lead to pitfalls that have been well documented in the relevant literature (Oppenheim, 1966). The layout of the questionnaire must be decided carefully. The presentation must be efficient and minimise the risk of errors. The data may be machine-processed; responses may need to be coded ready for computer analysis.

Problems may arise from differences between students in the way they respond to questionnaires, and precautions must be taken to reduce inaccuracies resulting from known limitations of respondents. For example, some students show a general tendency to agree rather than disagree with any statement presented; to counteract this tendency, some of the statements presented should be phrased positively while others should be phrased negatively. Again, many respondents use the middle point on any issue; a four-point scale will force them to commit themselves either against the statement or in favour of it.

Even in a study of attitudes, many items in the questionnaire need to be included simply to enquire about facts and actual behaviour. Facts such as age, sex, previous schooling, etc., can be used to classify a sample of respondents into subgroups for comparative analysis. Behavioural characteristics about which enquiry can be made include, for instance, the student's habits of study. However, the measurement of attitudes is more complex. Probing below the surface by indirect questions is often required (Bernstein, 1970), and this differentiates attitude study from behavioural inquiry. Attitude questioning is not only characterised by indirectness. Another factor is the complex way a person's attitudes are organised; a person may hold two sets of values which actually conflict with one another.

The items in a questionnaire are often written in a dichotomous form, respondents being required to select between two alternatives. A single item of this kind cannot be expected to disclose so complex an attribute as an attitude. Nor can a group of such questions provide insight into the way medical students feel, why they feel that way, and how they will feel and act in the future. A questionnaire may include a number of items which are not independent of each other, but overlap. By grouping the responses to such items, broader dimensions of attitude are discovered. It is often the underlying broad attitude dimension that is of interest to the investigator, rather than specific answers to individual items. Such combination of previously agreed groups of related questions may yield answers which can be used for the development of attitude scales.

Scales

Examples of two such scales, widely used in educational research, are the Complexity and the Thinking-Introversion scales of the Omnibus Personality Inventory.

The *Complexity (Co) Scale* consists of 27 items each exploring whether a person has an open-minded, experimental orientation rather than a fixed way of viewing events. Three items in the scale are the following:-
(a) Usually I prefer known ways of doing things rather than trying out new ways
(b) For most questions there is just one right answer, once a person is able to get all the facts
(c) I don't like to undertake any project unless I have a pretty good idea how it will turn out.
These items will be rejected by the high scorer, i.e. the complex person, who prefers diversity and is not uncomfortable in ambiguous situations; he is flexible and tolerant of unusual conditions. In contrast, the person who answers 'yes' to the above items, is a low scorer; he seeks definite structure and shuns unusual experiences. He dislikes circumstances which are novel or uncertain and he tends to be impatient with unfamiliar ideas.

The *Thinking-Introversion (TI) Scale* consists of 67 items. A high scorer inclines towards reflective thought and has a liking for abstract ideas. He will agree with such items as:-
(a) I study and analyse my own motives and reactions,
(b) When I go to a strange city I visit museums and galleries.
Among items he rejects is:-
(c) I am more realistic than idealistic, that is, more occupied with things as they are than with things as they should be.
This item is endorsed by the low scorer, the thinking-extravert, who customarily expresses practical ideas and prefers to act rather than to reflect. When exploring attitudes to psychiatry in senior medical students, high scores on the Co and TI scales are correlated with a positive attitude to the specialty, while low scorers have a negative attitude (Walton, 1967).

There is a statistical procedure, factor analysis, which can be used in the development of attitude scales. By this method, responses to questions are sorted into groups or 'factors' on the basis of the extent to which they are measuring common ground. The assumption is made that each item in the factor is measuring something in common, i.e. an underlying attitude dimension. The value of factor analysis in attitude scaling is that no previous assumptions are made about the precise nature of the attitude to be measured, or the degree of consistency between the items in any scale (Walton, 1968).

The wording of items in an attitude scale can take many forms. Two forms which can quantify the strength of an attitude are frequently chosen to assess students' attitudes. The *Likert Scale* was used, for example, by Eron (1955) in his study on the growth of cynicism (versus humanitarianism) in medical students. A student given items of Likert-type is asked to respond to pre-worded statements, different possibilities being presented; where he puts his tick indicates agreement or disagreement and the intensity with which the value is held. For example, in a study of 'cynical' attitudes a statement offered was 'Most people are out for what they can get'. The subject then responds on a five-point scale:-

    Strongly agree   5
    Agree   4
    No opinion   3
    Disagree   2
    Strongly disagree   1

The weights attached to each item are then added to give a total score. There are problems of interpretation of responses on a Likert scale. The student may wish to convey a socially favourable impression instead of responding frankly; such tendency to project an acceptable image compounds misreporting due to possible self-deception, the tendency to see oneself more favourably than others do. Furthermore, a verbal statement does not necessarily imply that the attitude expressed will be reflected in the student's actual behaviour.

The *Semantic Differential* (Osgood, Suci and Tannenbaum, 1957) is a form of diagrammatic scale which can be used to study a student's values and beliefs, his view of different medical specialists or specialties, teaching methods, types of patients, future career patterns, etc. The Semantic Differential allows the student to record his position in terms of bipolar opposites to statements presented. A seven-point scale is used, the 'good' value at one pole and the 'bad' at the other:-

    No   Yes

    1   2   3   4   5   6   7

For example, the statement 'Lecturer X was audible' can be presented at the end of a course. The student who checks at point 7 conveys an extreme positive rating (audible), while the student who places his check at point 1 indicates an extreme negative rating (inaudible).

Rating scales made up of such items can be used not only to investigate professional attitudes of medical students, but also their interests (Cowell and Entwistle, 1971), the values they hold, their study habits and their work preferences (Brown and Holtzman, 1966; Entwistle and Entwistle, 1970) and their views about the adequacy of their training. It is thus evident that they have particular application to in-course assessment in its monitoring role.

Simulated patients

Barrows (1971), as has been noted in Chapter 4, has done pioneer work in training housewives, secretaries or unemployed actors to simulate patients. This approach may be used to test the student's sensitivity and responsiveness to a patient's needs, as well as for the evaluation of purely clinical skills.

The response of a student to alternative lines of action offered in the course of a videotaped interview with a simulated awkward patient may also prove useful. The Department of Psychiatry in Birmingham is active in this field.

Another approach is the use of a role-playing doctor who, during the oral examination, assumes the role of a patient (Lamont and Hennen, 1972). The examiner then rates each candidate for specific aspects of the way the 'patient' is managed. For example:-
- (a) How effectively did he elicit the pertinent information?
- (b) Did he address the 'patient' in appropriate language?
- (c) Did he talk to the 'patient' in terms appropriate to his social class and his vocabulary?
- (d) Was he patronising? Did he talk too much? Did he listen?
- (e) Did he explain his plan of management in a sensible, rational way, which the 'patient' would be able to understand?

Once a set of criteria is defined, scores can be assigned and the 'affective domain' quantitatively explored. The examiner who takes part in a role-playing oral examination can be required to rate the candidate on numerical or diagrammatic scales, such as those described above, on specified clinical attitudes. For example:-
- (a) Does the candidate open the clinical interrogation satisfactorily?
- (b) Does he make you as a patient feel comfortable?
- (c) Does he align himself sufficiently sympathetically to grasp your problems?
- (d) Does he show more than casual interest in the social circumstances accompanying the particular problem you described?

The College of Family Physicians of Canada and the American Board of Orthopaedic Surgery both make regular use of this approach, though only rare and informal attention has been paid to it in Britain so far.

REFERENCES

Barrows, H.S. (1971) *Simulated Patients*. Springfield, Illinois: Charles C. Thomas.

Bernstein, L. (1970) Changes in 'Acceptance of Others' resulting from a course in the physician-patient relationship. *British Journal of Medical Education*, 4, 65.

Brown, W.F. and Holtzman, W.H. (1966) *Manual of Survey of Study Habits and Attitudes*. New York: The Psychological Corporation.

Charvat, J., McGuire, C. and Parsons, V. (1968) A Review of the Nature and Uses of Examinations in Medical Education. Geneva : World Health Organisation.

Cowell, M.D. and Entwistle, N.J. (1971) The relationships between personality, study attitudes and academic performance in a technical college. *British Journal of Educational Psychology*, 41, 85.

Entwistle, N.J. and Entwistle, D. (1970) The relationship between personality and academic performance. *British Journal of Educational Psychology*, 40, 132.

Eron, L.D. (1955) Effect of medical education on medical students' attitudes. *Journal of Medical Education*, 30, 559.

Flexner, A. (1930) *Universities, American, English, German*. London : Oxford University Press.

Lamont, C.T. and Hennen, B.K.E. (1972) The use of simulated patients in a certification examination in family medicine. *Journal of Medical Education*, 47, 789.

Levine, H.G. and McGuire, C. (1971) Rating habitual performance in graduate medical education. *Journal of Medical Education*, 46, 306.

Oppenheim, A.N. (1966) *Questionnaire Design and Attitude Measurement*. London : Heinemann.

Osgood, C.E., Suci, G.J. and Tannenbaum, P.H. (1957) *The Measurement of Meaning*. Illinois : University of Illinois Press.

Reitsma, F.E. (1973) *Human relations skills - training for medical students*. Division of Educational Development, Faculty of Medicine, University of Utrecht. Mimeograph: Association for Medical Education in Europe: Dundee.

Walton, H.J. (1967) The measurement of medical students' attitudes. *British Journal of Medical Education*, 1, 330.

Walton, H.J. (1968) Aims of teachers of psychiatry in five medical schools. *British Journal of Psychiatry*, 114, 1417.

6. Scoring

Whatever form an examination may take, it is necessary to describe the performance of the candidates in terms which can be understood by all concerned. Most commonly a numerical scale of marks is used but sometimes, particularly in the United States, students are classified into alphabetical grades. In disciplines other than medicine, the first three letters of the Greek alphabet have been used for this purpose, often embellished with plus and minus signs. One of us still recalls the symbols which recorded his attempts to produce Ciceronian Latin; the marks ranged, with incredible nicety, from the rarely achieved brilliance of α++ through grades such as β+?+ and β-, to the ignominy of γ--. Such sophistication has only been surpassed by computer marking of MCQ papers, in which candidates' percentage scores are commonly calculated to two places of decimals; the impressive range of 10,000 possible marks is thus obtained.

We have already emphasised how important it is, in the design of an examination, to define in advance the objectives of the exercise. This is no less important in the scoring. Most examinations in medicine consist of several parts, the scores in which are combined to produce a few grades such as Fail, Pass and, perhaps, one or more Honours Classes. From time to time, however, finer discrimination is required, particularly if useful feed-back to the candidates is to be provided. These factors and others, such as the proposed difficulty of the examination, should determine the scoring system to be employed.

When a numerical system is used, a pass mark is often required. This will be discussed in greater detail in relation to scoring MCQ papers but, in most subjectively scored examinations, a pass mark of 50 per cent is chosen. It has never been clear to us whether this is intended to imply that, in order to pass, a candidate is expected to know 50 per cent of what he is supposed to have learnt or 50 per cent of all the possible knowledge on the subject being examined. Neither seems very likely and, in practice, the time-honoured figure of 50 per cent is nothing more than a symbol for 'Pass'. This interchangeability of numbers and lettered or named grades is implicit in the opening paragraph of this chapter and will be discussed further in connection with the scoring of essays, orals and practical examinations.

Before proceeding to a discussion of the scoring of different types of examination, two technical terms applied to scoring systems in general must be defined. *Peer-* or *norm- referenced* scoring signifies that a candidate's performance is assessed in relation to that of the other candidates - his peers. (The term should not be confused with peer-rating which is the assessment of a candidate *by* his peers.) A *criterion referenced* scoring system is one in which candidates are assessed in relation to an external standard of performance set, usually, by the examiners. A priori, the latter system would seem to be preferable, especially in medical qualifying examinations but, as Mattson (1971) has pointed out, virtually all assessment in education is, in practice, peer-referenced. Few, if any, examiners are uninfluenced by the general standard of the papers they mark or of the candidates whom they meet in an oral examination.

SCORING IN THE COGNITIVE DOMAIN

In general terms a candidate can respond to any question, at any taxonomic level, in one of only three possible ways. His answer may be either correct, incorrect or, if he is totally ignorant of the subject, non-existent. The marks awarded by an examiner will depend, naturally, on the correctness or otherwise of the response and may well be weighted according to his conception of the importance of the knowledge being tested; a frank confession of ignorance will often be penalised less heavily than an incorrect answer especially if the latter reveals a dangerous misconception by the candidate. These principles can be made explicit in the marking of MCQ papers but, as will be shown, are also implicit in the scoring of any test in the cognitive domain.

Written tests

Multiple-choice questions. It must be stated firmly, at the outset of this discussion, that, whatever the scoring system employed, an MCQ paper can do no more than place the candidates in rank order in terms of their ability to answer that particular paper. Furthermore, although the rank orders produced by different scoring systems nearly always differ in detail, it is rarely possible to demonstrate any statistically significant difference between them. The choice of a scoring system, therefore, depends on factors such as the range of marks which is desired and the judgement of the examiners on the 'fairness' of the various systems. This judgement can be based partly, as will be shown, on probability theory but is also partly intuitive and, in the final analysis, always arbitrary.

A major consideration in the scoring of MCQs is the fact that it is possible for a candidate to score, sometimes quite heavily, by guesswork alone. Various systems have been devised which are said, by some, to compensate for the effect of guessing. This is not an accurate description of the operation of these systems, the effect of which is to discourage rather than, in any sense, to compensate for guessing. The essence of these procedures is the deduction of marks for incorrect answers, or 'counter-marking'.

The simplest form of MCQ is one in which a candidate is presented with a statement and is required to indicate whether he regards it as true or false. A direct extension of this type of question is the independent true-false type described in Chapter 3. In both these types the marking system depends on the number of options open to the candidate. For some years after the introduction of the independent true-false question in Britain, candidates were required to indicate their choice only of the correct completions on the answer sheet; it was assumed that those completions not indicated in this way were regarded by the candidate as false. He thus had two options only and was compelled to answer all the questions, some of them, perforce, by guesswork. If, with such questions, one mark is given for each completion correctly identified as true or false and zero for each incorrect identification (+1,0) a candidate who returned a blank answer sheet would automatically score as many marks as there were false completions in the paper; alternatively, by marking all the completions, he could score on all those which were true. Thus the range of all the candidates' marks, with such a marking system, is inevitably restricted to the upper end of the scale. The range of marks could be widened by counter-marking to the extent of deducting one mark for each incorrect answer (+1, -1) but this procedure would have no effect whatever on the rank order. The purpose of counter-marking is to discourage guessing by the candidates and it is therefore inappropriate when they are forced to guess by the very nature of the questions. The problem of the narrow range of marks is better solved by a system of scaling such as is discussed below.

Some complicated systems of counter-marking have been used in the past to score the type of independent true-false MCQ in which guessing is compelled. In one instance, for example (Study Group, 1967), the number of completions in each question varied from four to ten and the counter-marking was designed to ensure that the total possible score for each question was always the same. The formula used was $+1/p - 1/q$ where p was the number of correct completions and q the number of incorrect completions in the question. Thus a candidate obtained $1/p$ mark for each correct completion correctly indicated and $1/q$ was deducted for each incorrect completion marked by the candidate as true. The possible score for each question ranged from -1 to +1 and a candidate who marked all or none of the completions as true obtained no marks for that question. The main disadvantage of this and other similar systems (Buckley-Sharp and Harris, 1971) is that it introduces a sizeable weighting of the marks allotted to the various completions which depends on the relative numbers of correct and incorrect completions rather than on the importance of the knowledge being tested.

In recent years it has become customary, in several examinations, to increase the number of options open to the candidates in independent true-false questions to three. By suitable design of the answer sheets, a candidate can be required to mark each completion as either true or false or, by failing to mark it as either, he can tacitly admit his ignorance. Candidates can guess as much or as little as they choose and, to discourage this, some system of counter-marking becomes necessary (Fleming *et al.*, 1974).

Before considering some of the counter-marking systems which have been devised, it is instructive to imagine oneself in the position of a candidate faced by a paper of independent true-false questions. (It is worth mentioning, in passing, that candidates should always be fully informed about the scoring system which will be used. Ill-informed speculation about the use of counter-marks of uncertain magnitude improves neither the reliability of the examination nor the morale of the candidates.) Let us imagine, therefore, that the candidate knows that he will score one mark for each completion correctly indicated as true or false, that he will lose a mark for each completion incorrectly indicated and that he will score zero for each completion left unanswered; this scoring system may be abbreviated as $+1,0,-1$. He probably begins by answering, with some confidence, those completions of which he is certain he knows the correct answer. He then studies the remaining completions and finds some about which he is completely ignorant. These he will probably choose to leave unanswered, although, if he is a gambler, he may prefer to mark them at random. He is thus left with a number of completions which 'ring a bell' more or less loudly. His reaction to these will depend on his personality. If he is cautious, he may well leave most of them unmarked, whereas a bolder spirit is likely to 'play his hunches' and mark the completions as true or false accordingly. Such action, based on incomplete knowledge, can hardly be regarded as blameworthy by doctors accustomed to making clinical judgements of a similar nature. One of us (Sanderson, 1973) has studied the effect of candidates' personalities on their performance in this type of examination and has shown that the answer sheets of candidates whose performances in the examination ranged around the median for the class contained as many as 35 per cent or as few as 2 per cent of unmarked completions. This investigation also showed that reducing the counter-mark from 1 to 0.5 reduced the total unanswered completions from 18.1 per cent to 15.8 per cent, an unimpressive, though statistically significant, difference.

Lennox (1967) has approached the problem of determining the optimum value of a counter-mark from a statistical standpoint. He emphasised the need for the value to be large enough to be 'a sufficient deterrent' to guessing and suggested that -2 was appropriate. He illustrated the effect of this on the score of a candidate who could answer 50 out of 100 completions correctly and guessed the remainder; with a counter-mark of -2 he would improve on his 'true' mark of 50 less than once in 40 attempts. While we agree that this would be a powerful deterrent to guessing, it is our clear impression, obtained from informal discussion with many examination candidates, that, faced by the risk of such a penal mark, few would venture to answer any questions other than those about which they felt absolutely confident. Many candidates would thus be deprived of the opportunity of gaining credit for less than certain knowledge (Sanderson, 1973). Our personal preference is for the more modest counter-mark of -1 so that he who 'fears his fate too much', and there are many such, is more likely to do himself justice.

Another approach to the problem of counter-marking is confidence testing which has been proposed by Rothman (1969) and subsequently discussed by Paton (1971) and Palva and Korhonen (1973). With this system a candidate is required to indicate not only his choice of the correct completions but also the degree of confidence he has in his choice. Thus, he is asked to state, by marking an appropriate answer sheet, whether he is (a) very sure of his answer, (b) fairly sure, or (c) his answer is a guess. The scoring systems proposed by Rothman and by Paton are as follows:

Answer	*Confidence*	*Score*	
		Rothman	Paton
Correct	Very sure	+ 4/3	+ 5/3
	Fairly sure	+ 1	+ 4/3
	Guess	+ 2/3	+ 1
Incorrect	Guess	+ 1/3	- 1/3
	Fairly sure	0	- 1/2
	Very sure	- 1/3	- 1

One of the results of these marking systems is a range of candidates' marks wider than that obtained by conventional marking systems. This is not necessarily an advantage unless, at the same time, the rank order is made more 'correct', whatever that may mean. Although we have no personal experience of confidence testing, it seems to us that the 'confidence' of the candidates is likely to be greatly influenced by their personalities and by their interpretation of expressions such as 'fairly sure'. Furthermore, the selection of the most appropriate counter-marking system seems to pose further problems which are not easily solved. Of the two systems quoted, we would prefer Paton's as it gives no credit for an incorrect guess as does Rothman's. On the whole, as we have said, we favour equal marks and counter-marks although we accept that our liking for symmetry may be based on aesthetic rather than on scientific considerations.

Another matter which requires comment is the possibility of weighting the mark awarded for questions, or individual completions, according to the importance of the knowledge being tested. This is certainly done in subjectively scored tests and the possibility of rewarding accurate knowledge of an important subject or of penalising dangerous errors certainly has an appeal. However, our tentative efforts in this direction have foundered on our failure to obtain agreement among examiners on the relative importance of different questions. Dudley (1969) has recorded a similar experience. A more formal study of this problem is in progress (Sanderson and Fleming, to be published) and our preliminary results confirm that unanimity of opinion among medical men is the rare exception rather than the rule; few will be surprised at this finding.

We have discussed the scoring of the independent true-false MCQ at some length as we are most familiar with this type of question. However, many of our comments also apply, mutatis mutandis, to the current American formats discussed in Chapter 3. In these questions only one completion out of four or, more often, five, is correct and the candidate is awarded a mark for choosing that completion. Thus the question is scored as a whole unlike the independent true-false type in which, as the name implies, each completion is scored independently. Countermarking likewise must be applied to the question as a whole. We have already expressed our preference for the modest countermark of -1 for each incorrectly indicated completion of an independent true-false question; this is the mark which Lennox (1967) described as 'fair' i.e. that mark which allows candidates with the same amount of knowledge equal chances of scoring the same final mark. On this basis we would favour a countermark of -0.25 for an incorrect choice in a five-choice completion question or, in general terms, $-1/n-1$ where n is the number of possible answers to the question.

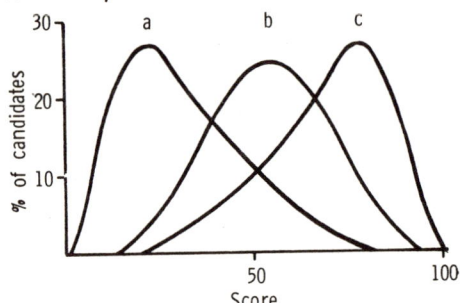

Fig. 1. *Theoretical frequency distributions of marks of candidates in (a) a difficult examination, (c) an easy examination and (b) most large public examinations in medicine.*

When a MCQ paper has been scored, the frequency distribution of the marks should be studied. Ideally this matter should have been considered at the time the objectives of the examination were defined. Thus it might be that the objective was to determine whether the candidates had mastered certain basic essential facts and principles; rather easy questions would be set and one would hope that a large majority of the candidates would score somewhere near the maximum possible mark. The resulting mark distribution would be strongly negatively skewed with a peak near the upper end and a tail extending in the direction of zero (Fig. 1c). By contrast, in an honours examination, the questions might well be so difficult that most of the candidates' scores would be in the lower end of the range and a positively skewed distribution would result (Fig.1a). In our experience, objectives are rarely defined with this degree of precision and it is, in any case, difficult to set an examination with a predetermined mark distribution without extensive pre-testing of the questions; this is rarely possible. In practice, in large public examinations, with most of the scoring systems in current use, a smooth unimodal distribution with a peak at, or a little above, 50 per cent is usually obtained (Fig. 1b). From such a distribution two distinct advantages accrue. The first is that its approximation to a normal or Gaussian form allows the valid use of standard statistics such as the mean and standard deviation. For example, from this information it is possible to calculate a series of *standard scores* from the expression $x/(\bar{x} - \sigma)$ where x is the candidate's mark, $\bar{x}$ is the mean of the distribution and σ is its standard deviation. This device is sometimes useful when the results of different examinations are being compared. Secondly. as will be shown in Chapter 7, the discriminating power of a paper, or of a single question, is at a maximum when the mean of the distribution, or the percentage of candidates correct, is 50 per cent. Difficulties arise with such a distribution, however, when it comes to setting the pass mark.

The range of marks obtained in a MCQ paper is usually wide and, except on the rare occasions when a rank order only is required, it is necessary to subdivide the candidates into a manageable number of groups by a scaling process. Various methods of scaling, which may be needed when a MCQ paper forms a part only of an examination, are discussed later in this chapter. Here we consider the simplest, yet the most important, scaling process in which candidates are divided into two groups only - Pass and Fail. This decision on the pass mark is most critical when the MCQ paper forms the whole examination.

One method which has been used occasionally is to study the frequency distribution of the marks for any suggestion of bimodality. This has nothing to recommend it as, even if the distribution were truly bimodal, which would be exceptional, there can be no assurance that the trough between the two peaks correctly represents the division between those who should pass and those who should fail. In any case, as we have said, the distribution is nearly always unimodal and, with large numbers, smooth, providing no intrinsic indication as to where the pass mark should be.

The approach to the problem of setting a fair pass mark can be on a basis of either criterion-reference or peer-reference. The concept of criterion-reference implies that there is a corpus of knowledge which a candidate *must* possess in order to pass. A paper set to test this basic knowledge will, of course, be very easy for most candidates; a negatively skewed mark distribution will be obtained and a pass mark near 90 per cent might well be set. This has the advantage of placing the pass mark on a section of the curve - the tail - where changes in its value will move the minimum number of candidates from the 'pass' to the 'fail' category or vice versa. The same argument applies to the positively skewed distribution resulting from a very difficult examination.

In practice, a rather strict peer-referenced system is quite widely employed so that the proportion of candidates passing an examination held regularly varies little from one occasion to the next. Many examiners, who are more familiar with scoring essay questions, feel that this arbitrary procedure is a serious disadvantage of MCQ and other objective examination methods. There is no doubt that the scoring of essays is criterion-referenced but, as we have shown, there are, unfortunately, as many criteria as there are examiners. A peer-referenced pass mark need not be quite as arbitrary as it might seem to be and can, or should, be modified by reference to certain indirect external criteria. It is, for example, common knowledge that, in large traditional examinations with several hundred candidates at a time, the proportion of candidates passing has not varied a great deal over the years. The passing of a similar proportion of candidates, taking a MCQ paper at a comparable stage of their course, would seem not unreasonable. The consistent behaviour of large groups of candidates can be made use of in another way. We, and others, have found that when a multiple-choice question is used on two separate occasions in an examination taken by several hundred candidates the mean scores of the two groups of candidates are very constant, often to within less than 1 per cent. It is, therefore, possible to include a few such 'marker' questions in a paper and to conclude that, if the candidates' scores on these questions remain constant, the average ability of the whole group of candidates is of the same order as on previous occasions. In that case, if the mean score of the candidates on the test as a whole were unusually high or low, it would be reasonable to infer that the test had, inadvertently, been made more easy or more difficult than usual. A pass mark which is some function of the mean score can then be used. The scatter of the marks should also be considered and it is quite common practice to set a pass mark at some multiple or fraction of the standard deviation away from the mean. With the near-normal distributions which are commonly seen the result, once more, is a fairly constant pass rate.

It must be freely admitted, however, that the decision on where to place the pass mark in terms of the mean and standard deviation, or of any other statistics of the score distribution, remains arbitrary and can only be made on the basis of the agreed purpose of the test. It is the function of some tests to exclude a higher proportion of candidates than others and the decision must be taken with this consideration in mind.

Other objective techniques. Under this heading we include all questions requiring answers consisting of one or two words or, at most, a phrase. Acceptable answers must have been agreed beforehand, as described in Chapter 3. Two aspects of the scoring of these questions require consideration. The first is the preliminary allocation of marks to the answers which have been anticipated. This process is criterion-referenced, the criteria being based on the collective experience of the examiners setting the questions and it is usually possible to obtain a fair degree of unanimity on the marks to be allotted. A seven-point scale of marks has proved satisfactory in our experience. A much wider or much narrower range than this may create difficulties for those who have to score the candidates' answers and allot marks, after brief consideration, to answers which had not been foreseen. The unanimity reached on the allocation of marks to these questions is to be contrasted with its conspicuous absence when the weighting of MCQs according to their importance is under consideration. This is almost certainly due to the fact that, in the latter case, examiners are required to make a value-judgement on, for example, the relative importance of the biochemical findings in cystinuria and the physical signs of obstructive cardiomyopathy. In the case of the tests under consideration, the point at issue is usually whether or not a particular diagnosis or method of management is more likely to be 'correct' than another and it is reasonable to expect experienced examiners to reach agreement on this. Indeed, it would be possible, for many such questions, to produce an extremely accurate scoring system based on conditional probability using Bayes' formula (Cliffe, 1968); we would not particularly recommend this practice but mention it to demonstrate that the problem of scoring such questions may be capable of precise solution.

The process of scaling the marks for such questions and of setting a pass mark, when necessary, is similar to that for MCQs. A criterion-referenced system could probably be devised but this, again, would involve difficult value-judgements and it is likely that peer-referenced systems will continue to be used.

It seems appropriate to comment briefly, here, on the scoring of Patient Management Problems (PMPs). We have no personal experience of this but it seems likely that, once a problem has been set - a task of no little difficulty - it should be possible to obtain agreement on the acceptability of candidates' responses. The end-result of a PMP is the improvement or death of the imaginary patient and criterion-based scoring should present little difficulty. The setting of a pass mark, however, involves macabre consideration of the maximum number of lethal mistakes a doctor may make and yet still be allowed to practise.

Essay questions. The marking of essay questions differs from that of objective questions in two ways. Firstly it is essentially criterion-referenced although, as we have said, with criteria varying with the views of the individual examiners. Secondly, the so-called close-marking system is often used so that the range of possible marks is small. This deliberate restriction of the range may be a conscious or subconscious recognition that the reliability of essay questions is poor and ensures that candidates can be neither penalised heavily nor unduly rewarded by marks whose accuracy is suspect.

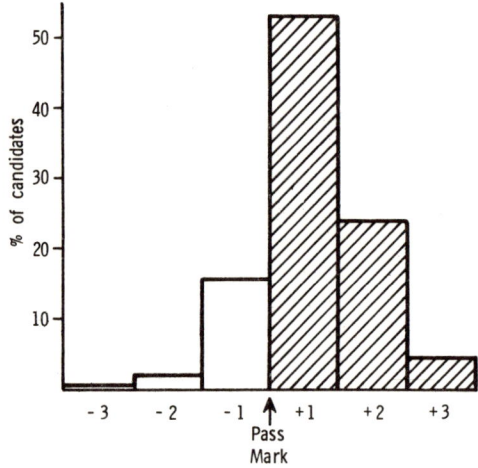

Fig. 2. Histogram of marks obtained by 854 candidates in the essay paper of a series of qualifying examinations in medicine. The hatched area represents the candidates who obtained a mark higher than the pass mark.

The narrow range itself also ensures that attempts to improve the discriminatory power of such questions can have only limited success. In practice the range of marks is often narrowed still further by many examiners who, perhaps influenced by widespread criticism of essay questions, are unwilling to trust their judgement and prefer to use the middle of the range only. This is illustrated in Figure 2 which shows the distribution of the marks allotted in 854 essay papers in a series of qualifying examinations in medicine. The numbers of candidates scoring each of the six possible marks is expressed as a percentage of the whole and it will be seen that 0.12 per cent i.e. one candidate, was given the lowest possible mark and a further 2.34 per cent received the next lowest. The process is, in fact, no longer scoring but has been converted into grading. The only valid reason for retaining numerical values for the marks is the need, in many examinations, to combine the marks of different parts to obtain a total. The difficulties which arise when this is done are discussed below.

There is no simple solution to the problem of marking essay questions but it seems to us that the existing systems might be improved in two ways. The first is the elimination of the variability of the criteria by which the candidates' answers are judged and the second is the use of a wider, and therefore more discriminating, range of marks. One approach is to arrange that each paper is marked by several examiners, perhaps four or even six, working independently and with no knowledge of the marks awarded by their colleagues. Averaging the marks of all the examiners would automatically result in a wider range, measured in terms of the number of points on the scale. It also seems probable that the effect of variable criteria would be reduced and there is evidence that the reliability of essay questions marked in this way is fairly high. However, few examiners would welcome a proposal that they should mark six times as many essay papers as they do at present and this system would be unacceptable except, perhaps, in examinations with very few candidates. A more profitable, although not necessarily less time-consuming, system has been mentioned in Chapter 3. This involves detailed preliminary consideration by the examiners of the probable content of the candidates' essays. Agreement would have to be reached on the points which would be required in an acceptable essay and on the marks to be allotted to each of these points. In this way, agreed criteria and a fairly wide range of marks are ensured. A similar method could be adopted, perhaps rather more easily, if the long traditional essays were replaced by a large number of shorter essays. It seems as reasonable to expect a candidate to be able to demonstrate his power of logical reasoning and original thought in an answer of 500 words as in one of 1500. Freeman and Byrne (1973) have described their successful use of such short essay questions and, despite our distrust of essay questions in general, we would favour further experiments along these lines.

Oral examinations

We have already made clear our view that the attributes currently tested in oral examinations can be assessed more reliably by other methods and that there seems to be no logical reason for retaining the oral examination as a means of testing in the cognitive domain. In this section, therefore, we propose to do no more than describe what seem to be the current methods of scoring oral examinations and to analyse a few of the extraneous factors which may influence the marks awarded.

As with essay questions, marking is criterion-referenced modified, we suspect, by a tendency to award a higher or lower mark to a candidate of average ability if he is examined after a series of very poor or very good candidates. The closemarking system is almost invariably used although examiners seem to make rather more use of the extremes of the range than with essay questions (Fig. 3). This may be due to the fact that there is very little time for deliberation before a mark is awarded and there is probably heavy weighting of the questions as examiners can hardly avoid being unduly influenced by the sudden fleeting exposure of a large gap in a candidate's knowledge or by a sudden flash of brilliance. As in the case of essay questions the numerical marks are no more than symbols for a series of grades.

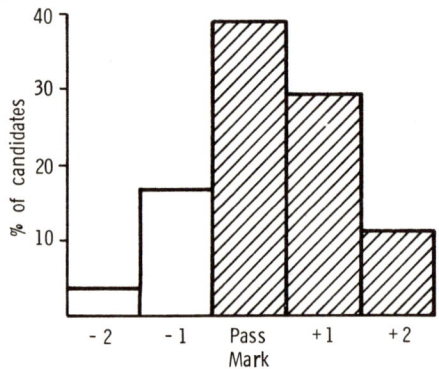

Fig. 3. Histogram of marks obtained by 854 candidates in the oral sections of a series of qualifying examinations in medicine. The hatched area represents the candidates who obtained a pass mark or higher.

Among the factors influencing the marking of oral examinations is the effect a pair of examiners have upon each other. We have shown (Fleming *et al.*, 1974) that when a candidate is examined by two pairs of examiners and each of the examiners records his mark independently, the marks of two examiners sitting together are closely correlated but have no significant correlation with the marks given by the other pair. The fluctuating benevolence of examiners is another factor although it is difficult to quantify. The mythology of examinations includes a widely-held belief that examiners give higher marks after they have had their coffee; as Richard Gordon's Old Stager said 'A low blood sugar is conducive to bad temper' (Gordon, 1952). We have not been able to substantiate this but have, in fact, noticed an interesting and not wholly explicable, tendency for examiners to give higher marks just before lunch. Figure 4 shows the distributions of oral marks given to the first and last candidates during a series of oral examinations, held in the mornings. There is a clear tendency to award the highest possible mark much more often at the end of the morning than at the beginning. The difference between the two distributions is statistically significant ($\chi^2 = 30.1$; $p < 0.001$).

SCORING IN THE PSYCHOMOTOR DOMAIN

Practical laboratory examinations

We have no personal experience in this area and do not feel competent to make more than a few general comments. It seems likely that the scoring systems employed depend on whether the examiner is assessing the candidate's manual dexterity and is thus testing strictly within the psychomotor domain or whether he is trying to draw inferences, from the candidate's actions, about his understanding of the subject in question. In the former case, an accurate criterion-referenced assessment would be quite practicable as the end-result of a practical examination will often be either a tangible object such as a stained slide or the numerical result of a physical or chemical experiment. There should be little difficulty in defining stable and constant criteria for the assessment of such results and this is probably also the case if the candidate's dexterity in handling laboratory equipment is also being judged. When it comes to drawing inferences about a candidate's understanding of a problem, we would suspect, from our experience as clinical examiners, that, as with other subjectively scored examinations, criteria fluctuate and vary from examiner to examiner.

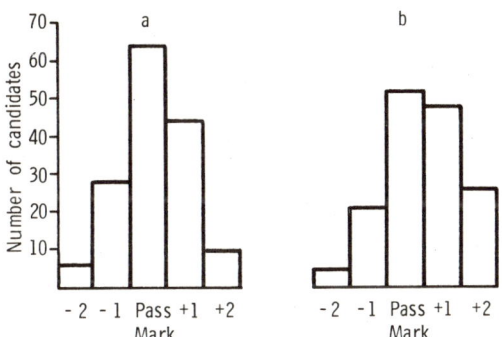

Fig. 4. Histograms of marks obtained by (a) those candidates who were examined first and (b) those who were examined last in a series of oral examinations held in the mornings.

Clinical examinations

In practically all undergraduate and postgraduate examinations the 'clinical' is the one part in which a failure cannot be compensated for by excellence in other parts. This fact has an important influence on the scoring. It might have been thought that all that was required was a series of marks, or, more correctly, grades with numerical symbols, including Fail,

Pass and Pass plus one or more bonus marks to compensate for possible failure in other parts of the examination. In practice the close-marking range which is usually prescribed is distributed equally on either side of the pass mark and a special convention may be adopted to allow for the reluctance of examiners, well aware of the imperfections of the examination, to make the crucial pass/fail decision with little time for deliberation. Figure 5 shows the distribution of marks obtained in the clinical part of a qualifying examination and several points should be noted. The first is the sizeable number of

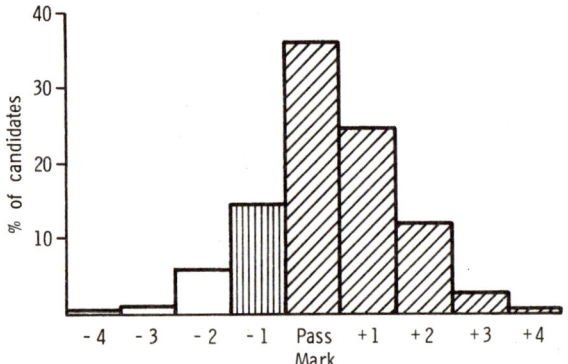

Fig. 5. *Histogram of marks obtained by 854 candidates in the clinical sections of a series of qualifying examinations in medicine. The diagonally hatched area represents the candidates who obtained a pass mark or higher; the vertically hatched area represents those candidates who did not satisfy the examiners but did, nevertheless, not fail irredeemably.*

candidates who have scored Pass -1; these have just failed to satisfy the examiners but will often, by convention, be given an extra mark in the 'clinical' if they have passed the remainder of the examination. A mark of Pass -2 denotes irredeemable failure. Pass -3 and Pass -4 have the same significance and are therefore redundant grades except perhaps as a means of allowing examiners to relieve their feelings about a candidate's abysmal incompetence. There are thus effectively two grades of failure - Certain Fail and Possible Fail and five pass grades. The system is probably reasonably equitable in the context of a criterion-referenced subjective scoring system but could almost certainly be improved by preliminary precise definition of criteria as in the case of essay questions. The application of this principle to clinical examinations has been discussed in Chapter 4.

SCORING A WHOLE EXAMINATION

Most examinations in medicine consist of several parts

including, for example, essay and MCQ papers with oral and clinical (or practical) examinations. If that is the case, a decision has to be made on the proportions of the total marks to be allotted to each part. A commonly used ratio of marks for clinical : written paper : oral is of the order 3:2:1 and this might well be expressed as totals of 150, 100 and 50. It is important to realise, however, that it is not the theoretical maximum possible marks but the few marks in the middle of the range which the examiners actually use which determine the relative weights of the different parts. Thus, if the examiners confine their marking to a five-point scale for each part, and this is quite common practice, they nullify the effect of the weighting system.

Particular problems arise when one of the parts of an examination is a MCQ paper which, as we have said, produces a rank order of candidates; the combination of this with the series of grades used in most other parts of an examination requires a great deal of careful thought. There is, in fact, no really satisfactory method of combining marks obtained by peer-reference with those resulting from a criterion-referenced system. In practice, to reconcile the normally distributed MCQ marks with the narrow ranges of marks of other parts which usually have a more or less negatively skewed distribution, some form of non-linear scaling of the former is necessary. Having been asked on several occasions to advise on scaling systems for various examinations, we propose to discuss the matter in some detail if only to demonstrate our own uncertainty. We are well aware how easy it is to distort the result of a whole examination by an unwise choice of scaling system.

Scaling of MCQ marks

The first, and most critical, step is to decide on the appropriate form of the distribution of scaled marks. This involves a process similar to that which was discussed earlier in this chapter in connection with setting a pass mark on a MCQ paper. Our own practice is to obtain as much information as possible about the marks obtained in the parts of previous examinations which were used for testing in the cognitive domain; it has, so far, always been the case that a MCQ paper has been introduced into established examinations and the requisite information has been available. If the marks of several hundred candidates are available, a reasonably smooth frequency distribution can be constructed with the close-marking range which has been used on the abscissa. It then becomes possible to determine the proportions of candidates who have received each of the marks in the range. All that remains is to decide on the most appropriate mathematical manipulation to be applied to the raw MCQ marks so as to produce the same distribution of marks. One approach is similar to that suggested for the determination of the pass mark, using various functions of the mean and fractions of the standard deviation of the raw MCQ mark distribution as scaling factors. If study of the marks of previous examinations has revealed that the standard deviation has been fluctuating significantly without much change in the mean mark, it may be preferable to use a simpler version of this system in which the fractions of the standard deviation are replaced by absolute numbers of marks derived from a standard deviation calculated from many previous examinations. A third system, which we favour at present, involves the use of percentile marks. In this, the actual MCQ marks are discarded and the scaling is based on the rank order only. The percentile mark is calculated from the expression $(100/N) \times (N+1-r)$ where N is the total number of candidates and r the rank position of the candidate in question. We have found that some examiners are unfamiliar with the concept of percentile marks and one or two examples may be helpful. If there were exactly 100 candidates, the candidate who headed the rank order (and whose rank position was therefore 1) would have a percentile mark of 100. For 300 candidates the candidate who stood 62nd in the rank order would have a percentile mark of $(100/300) \times (300+1-62) = 79.67$

The advantages of this system are firstly that it is the rank order generated by a MCQ paper which is the most accurate measure of the performances of the candidates and secondly that it is easy to produce a mark-distribution virtually identical to that of previous examinations. By this means a violent change in the pass-rate of an examination, resulting from the introduction of a MCQ paper, can be avoided. One final point should be made. We have shown that examiners are often reluctant to use the whole of the prescribed range of marks and it must be remembered that, however the MCQ marks are scaled, they will automatically be spread over the whole of the possible range and may, therefore, when combined with the marks of other parts, have a disproportionate effect on the result of the examination as a whole. Whether or not this is desirable is debatable but it is certainly important to recognise that it will occur unless an appropriate reduction in the range of the scaled MCQ marks is made.

The profile system

Having outlined current practice in marking examinations with several parts and indicated a few ways in which minor improvements could be made, we believe that the time has come when a critical study should be made of this process in which, with the exception of the 'clinical', it is possible to compensate for a poor performance in one part of an examination by a good mark in another. The relationship between separate parts can be studied in several ways. If the mark-distributions are normal, or nearly so, the correlation coefficient between any two sets of marks can be calculated. If this is found to be significant, it is sometimes regarded as evidence that the examination as a whole is reliable. It could, however, equally well be an indication that the two parts are assessing the same attributes and that one of the parts is redundant. If, on the other hand, the marks of two parts are not significantly correlated and provided, of course, that the reliability of each part is satisfactory, it is reasonable to infer that different attributes are being tested. We have already emphasised the importance, in the design of an examination, of defining the essential attributes to be possessed by successful candidates and then subdividing the examination into as many parts, each perhaps with several subsections, as are needed to test those attributes. With the wealth of detailed information about candidates resulting from such an examination, it seems a pity arbitrarily to aggregate the marks of all the parts, thereby implying that some of the attributes are not really essential provided that a candidate possesses others in full measure. The process is no more sensible than making a cake with double the amount of butter to compensate for a shortage of flour. We suggest that, provided an examination has been properly designed, it is reasonable to require a candidate to obtain a pass mark, at whatever level that may be set, in all the parts and to demonstrate thereby that he possesses all the attributes which are considered necessary. This is known as the 'profile' system.

REFERENCES

Buckley-Sharp, M.D. and Harris, F.T.C. (1971) The scoring of multiple-choice questions. *British Journal of Medical Education*, 5, 279.
Cliffe, P. (1968) Computers in medicine. In *Recent Advances in Medicine*, 15th edition, ed. Baron, D.N., Compston, N. and Dawson, A.M. Ch.1. London : Churchill.
Dudley, H.A.F. (1969) Objects of objective tests : a theoretical and experimental analysis. *British Journal of Medical Education*, 3, 155.
Fleming, P.R., Manderson, W.G., Matthews, M.B., Sanderson, P.H. and Stokes, J.F. (1974) Evolution of an examination : M.R.C.P. (U.K.). *British Medical Journal*, 1, 99.
Freeman, J. and Byrne, P.S. (1973) *The assessment of post-graduate training in general practice*. London : Society for Research into Higher Education.
Gordon, R. (1952) *Doctor in the house*. London : Michael Joseph.
Lennox, B. (1967) Marking multiple-choice examinations. *British Journal of Medical Education*, 1, 203.
Mattson, D.E. (1971) Criterion related measures in education. *Journal of Medical Education*, 46, 185.
Palva, I.P. and Korhonen, V. (1973) Confidence testing as an improvement of multiple-choice examinations. *British*

Journal of Medical Education, 7, 179.
Paton, D.M. (1971) An examination of confidence testing in multiple-choice examinations. *British Journal of Medical Education*, 5, 53.
Rothman, A.I. (1969) Confidence testing : an extension of multiple-choice testing. *British Journal of Medical Education*, 3, 237.
Sanderson, P.H. (1973) Prediction of student performance by multiple choice testing. *British Journal of Medical Education*, 7, 251.
Study Group of the Royal College of Physicians of London (1967) Experience of multiple-choice-question examination for Part I of the M.R.C.P. *Lancet*, 2, 1034.

7. Analysis of Results

In the past, there seems to have been a feeling that once an examination had yielded a rank-order of candidates or a pass-list, the examiner's work was done. Little or no attempt was made to find out whether or not the test had achieved what was intended. With the development of objective techniques yielding detailed scores, and the availability of computers, important new information, about the tests rather than about the candidates, has begun to emerge. The impact of this on the design of the tests has been striking. Modification of test material in the light of these results has greatly improved its effectiveness (Fleming et al., 1974) and has thrown unexpected light on the way in which it functions; it is becoming clear that this is a process which should be applied to all tests, whether objective or not.

The information emerging from this process, generally known as 'item analysis', relates to four main attributes of the item or of the whole test: difficulty, discriminating power, reliability and validity.

DIFFICULTY

The difficulty of an examination, or of an item which is part of it, is easy enough to determine for that particular group of candidates; for a whole test or for a question relating to several completions, the mean score is required, while for an individual completion, the percentage of candidates giving the correct response is appropriate. Such information is very easily obtained through a computer. It must be interpreted in the light of the stage of instruction which the candidates have reached. Being derived from a finite number of candidates, the results are subject to ordinary statistical variation; they represent a sample of the ideal population of all candidates who have reached that particular stage. The actual scores of a group of candidates will be spread out over a range, and while the resulting frequency distribution is not always normal in form, it is usually sufficiently close to this for conventional statistical methods to be useful. Thus, we may calculate the mean and the standard deviation, and from this the standard error. If now we compare the mean scores of two groups of candidates for the same question, we are in a position (after the necessary calculations) to say what is the probability that the difference between them could be accounted for by chance alone. As a matter of observation, when successive groups of candidates at the same stage of training answer the same question, the mean score and the percentage giving correct responses usually show surprisingly little change. This finding has an important corollary - namely that if two groups of substantial size (say over 200) at the same stage of training sit two *different* examinations and the mean scores of the groups differ substantially, this is more likely to be due to differing standards of difficulty in the two examinations than to variation in ability between the two groups.

The level of difficulty to be aimed at for an item or for a whole test is determined mainly by educational considerations, as we have indicated in Chapter 6. However, when the test is required to produce the maximum discrimination between the candidates, it can be shown that the optimum difficulty of an item is that which allows 50 per cent of the candidates to answer it correctly. Suppose that we have an entry of 100 candidates, and that 50 of these make a correct response to a certain item. Each candidate making a correct response is thereby shown to be better informed than 50 others who made an incorrect response. The number of comparisons is thus 50 x 50 = 2500. Suppose now that another item is answered correctly by 90 candidates and incorrectly by 10. Ninety candidates are shown to be better informed than 10 others: the number of comparisons is only 900. Put mathematically, the number of comparisons is pq, where p is the number making a correct response and q the remainder. The value of pq reaches its maximum when p = q.

Where discrimination between individuals is the main purpose of the test, 50 per cent is clearly the optimum proportion of correct responses, and very easy and very difficult items will be less effective in this respect. The objectives of the test may dictate otherwise, however. In very easy or very difficult tests such as we have discussed in Chapter 6, the value of pq will be low for most items, but the discrimination will be taking place at the level where it is needed - among the bottom or the top 10 per cent of the class.

DISCRIMINATING POWER

By this we mean the effectiveness whereby an item distinguishes between able and less able candidates. The difficulty lies in the operational definition of these two categories. Some criterion of ability, such as the candidates' subsequent success or failure in their careers, would be ideal, although clearly this is impracticable. The criterion most commonly used, because of the ease with which it can be applied, is the candidate's performance in the test as a whole. Looking at it in another way, we might say that the best estimate we have of the candidate's educational status at the time is his performance in the whole test; the better this is reflected in his performance on a single item, the more accurately does this item assign him to his appropriate rank in the class. This approach is only acceptable if we can be reasonably sure that the test as a whole is in fact asking the right sort of questions.

It will be assumed in the following discussion that this internal criterion is in fact the one to be used in calculating discriminating power. The mathematics required is that of correlation and for those seeking more detailed information an excellent account is given by Guilford (1965). For our purposes, only two sets of conditions for correlation between item scores and total scores need be considered. In both cases the total scores may be treated as a continuous variable; the first case then is that of the single item, when the score may be 0 or 1, and the second case is the composite question involving several completions, where the score, being the sum of the scores of the individual completions, may again be regarded as continuously variable. The second case is in some ways the simpler, since it involves more familiar statistical methods, and will therefore be considered first.

The product-moment correlation coefficient

The appropriate statistic to be calculated is the Pearson, or product-moment, correlation coefficient. (Note however that for this coefficient to be valid both distributions must be unimodal. This leads to special problems with the +1, 0, -1 type of scoring for individual completions, as will be seen below). For directions as to the method of computing Pearson's r, as it is usually known, the reader is referred to any standard statistical text. Computation by hand, or even with a mechanical calculator, is laborious; for numbers up to about 100 a programmed electronic calculator is satisfactory but for anything much more than this a computer is needed.

A question which yielded a correlation coefficient of +1.0 would arrange the candidates in exactly the same rank order as that resulting from the total marks in the test. A coefficient of zero would imply that the scores on that question bore no relation whatever to the scores for the whole test. A negative coefficient would indicate that candidates who scored high marks in the whole test were scoring low marks on that question, and vice versa. From our point of view (subject to the reservations mentioned above about the test as a whole being composed of questions which are appropriate) what is needed is the highest possible value of r.

If two variables which in fact are completely independent of one another are the subject of a finite number of observations it is possible that, simply by chance, a correlation coefficient differing from zero will be obtained. The larger the number of observations the greater is the probability that an observed correlation is due to a real interdependence of the variables rather than to chance. If we apply this reasoning to a test, then the number of observations is the number of candidates and it is possible to calculate, for any such number, what values (positive or negative) r must reach before the likelihood of chance as an explanation can be discarded. The conventional level at which an observed correlation is first taken seriously is when the chance of it occurring fortuitously has fallen to 1 in 20, that is a probability of 0.05 (P = 0.05). Another conventional level, this time for 'highly significant' departure from zero, is P = 0.01 - a chance of 1 in 100. Some examples of the actual values of r required for 'significance' in these terms are shown below:

Number of Candidates	P = 0.05	P = 0.01
10	0.632	0.765
50	0.279	0.360
500	0.088	0.115

The importance of the number of candidates in assessing significance is obvious.

Questions yielding 'barely significant' correlation coefficients are, however, still some way from the best that can be achieved. With 500 candidates, the coefficients would need to be of the order of +0.3 before an experienced test committee would be much impressed, and values of +0.6 have been achieved. For small numbers of candidates the r values need to be much higher to give the same levels of significance, e.g. for 50 candidates a value as high as 0.93 is required to achieve the same significance as one of 0.6 for 500 candidates. The required information for candidate numbers between 50 and 500 is presented in graphical form in appendix A.

Despite this large area of uncertainty when the number of candidates is low, no difficulty need result provided that the need for much higher values of r for equivalent discriminating power under these circumstances is clearly recognised. A corollary of this effect, which also needs stressing, arises when the performance of a question in two successive tests is being studied. Suppose that in an examination involving 500 candidates a particular question yields an r of +0.30. In another examination the same question is used unaltered, and this time the r is +0.40. Has a significant change occurred, or could this have happened by chance? Use of the appropriate statistical test shows that such a difference could have happened by chance on 8 occasions out of 100 and therefore (using the conventional level of 5 per cent, P = 0.05) is statistically 'not significant'. A small further increase in the second observed r to +0.41 brings the probability down to below 0.05 and this difference would therefore be accounted 'significant'. With smaller numbers, however, much greater changes can occur in observed r values by the operation of chance alone. If we have an entry of only 100 candidates in both examinations, an r of +0.30 on the first occasion could rise to +0.53 or fall to

+0.03 on the second occasion without conventional 'significance' (P<0.05) being reached. Experience confirms these calculations, in that with candidate numbers of 100 and below, great variations in observed r values for the same question used on several occasions do in fact occur. With entries of this size attempts to improve a question in the light of its observed item-to-total correlation are seldom profitable on the basis of one observation only. When a particular question, or a completion within a question, is seen to have failed for the second or third time, the experimental basis for discarding the whole question or altering the unsatisfactory completion becomes stronger.

Another consideration in interpreting an observed r value derives from the influence of the difficulty of the question on the number of discriminations it can make (see above, p.68). As we have shown, very difficult questions exercise their discriminating power only among the top 10 per cent of the candidates, likewise very easy questions operate only among the least well-informed. There may, as we have suggested, be perfectly valid educational reasons why we should wish to produce discrimination among the members of these groups; on the other hand, when such conditions do not obtain, a question with an r of +0.30 which is answered correctly by 50 per cent of the candidates may well be just as effective, perhaps more so, than one with an r of +0.50 which was correctly answered by only 1 per cent.

We have considered the problems of interpreting Pearson's r in some detail because the same problems arise with the other correlation indices to be described below, and because in our experience examiners who are unaware of these limitations are apt to be unduly influenced by the magnitude of r (or of the equivalents) when reviewing questions in the light of the item analysis. In many cases the mean score or the percentage of correct answers may carry information which is just as important as the correlation index, or even more important, and yet there is a strong tendency for these to be ignored and for decisions about deletion of a question or alteration of a completion to be based on the correlation index alone, without any consideration as to how much confidence may be placed in the latter.

The point-biserial correlation coefficient

We must now consider corresponding tests for use with single completions, to which the candidates' response can be either correct or incorrect, scoring usually 1 or 0. One such index is the point-biserial correlation coefficient (r_{pbi}). There are good mathematical reasons for using it in this particular situation, but computer programmers have probably also been attracted to it by reason of a specially convenient feature; if a program for calculating Pearson's r is employed and the values 1 (for a correct response) and 0 (for an incorrect response) are entered as one variable together with the candidates' scores in the whole test as the other variable, then a point-biserial correlation coefficient emerges. It is also possible to test the significance of the difference between an observed r_{pbi} and zero with the same formula as that used for Pearson's r. Statistical treatment of the difference between two point-biserial correlation coefficients is complex; the formula applicable to the Pearson r can be used as a guide, but not too much confidence should be placed in the result.

Calculation of r_{pbi} by hand is laborious; the formula is therefore not given since, if a computer were not available, one of the two indices to be mentioned below, requiring simpler calculations, would be used.

The Φ coefficient

The Φ coefficient is the more widely used and more familiar of these. Its use involves the discarding of some of the information and it is therefore less reliable than r and r_{pbi}. However, it is this simplification of procedure which makes it so convenient to use if a computer is not available. The marks for the whole test are used, not as the continuous variable required for r and r_{pbi}, but as a means of arranging the candidates in rank order. The group can then be divided on the basis of this rank order into two equal (or nearly equal, if there is an odd number of candidates) sub-groups - an upper half and a lower half. Under these conditions of equal sub-groups, the formula for the Φ coefficient simplifies to

$$\Phi = \frac{p_u - p_l}{2\sqrt{pq}}$$

where p_u is the proportion of candidates in the upper half answering the completion correctly, p_l is the corresponding proportion for the lower half, p is the proportion for all candidates together and q is 1 - p. With the aid of tables for $\sqrt{pq}$, such as table G in Guilford (1965) Φ can be calculated easily and quickly with a slide-rule.

The convenience of Φ is its strongest asset. It has certain drawbacks which must be made clear, although they do not seriously hinder its use provided they are recognised. Firstly, its range is more or less limited as p departs from 0.5. Take the ideal case in which all the candidates in the upper half answer a completion correctly, and all in the lower half answer incorrectly. Then

$$\Phi = \frac{1.00 - 0}{2\sqrt{0.5 \times 0.5}} = 1.00$$

Suppose now that only half the candidates in the upper group answer correctly, while all the lower group answer incorrectly as before. Then

$$\Phi = \frac{0.5 - 0}{2\sqrt{0.25 \times 0.75}} = \frac{0.5}{2 \times 0.433} = 0.577$$

The completion is clearly acting in the most effective manner possible in separating the able candidates from the less able, in that all those who answered correctly are included in the upper half. Yet the value of Φ cannot be greater than 0.577. The same would be the case if only 25 per cent of the candidates answered incorrectly and all were in the lower half. If p rises to say 0.9 (or falls to 0.1) the maximum possible Φ falls to 0.333 (Fig. 6).

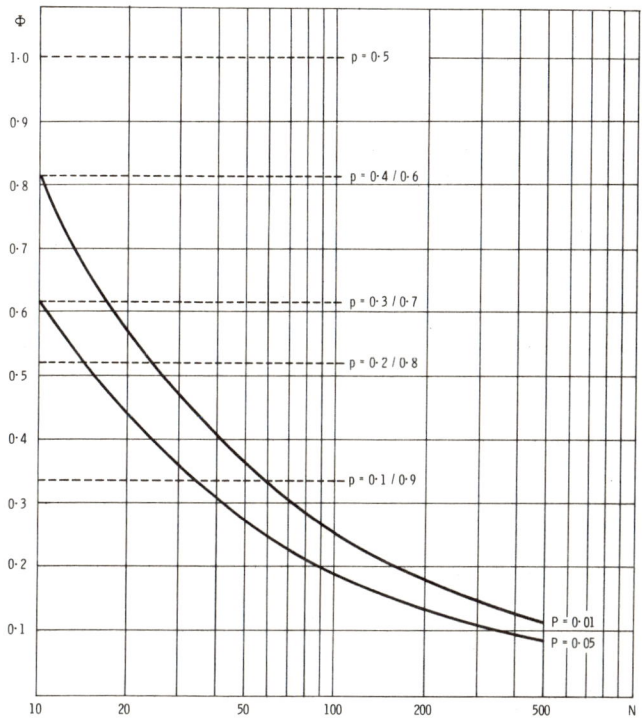

Fig. 6. Relationship between numbers of candidates (N) and values of Φ required for significance at the 5 per cent and 1 per cent levels (heavy curved lines). The horizontal dotted lines represent the maximum possible values of Φ for questions of given difficulty.

In actual practice this limitation of Φ seldom causes serious problems, but its existence should be borne in mind. In one sense it may be valuable; we have already seen that a question or completion which is very easy or very difficult exerts its discriminatory power on fewer candidates than one which is of median difficulty. The limitation of the range of Φ gives some expression to this.

The Φ coefficient has another limitation, similar to that of the point-biserial correlation coefficient; calculation of its standard error is extremely laborious and so the comparison, on a statistical basis, between two observed values of Φ is not often feasible. Reference to a standard statistical text will show that, if N = the number of candidates, $N\Phi^2 = \chi^2$. From this relationship the corresponding value of χ^2 can be calculated and tables of the distribution of χ^2 for one degree of freedom will show the probability of the chance occurrence of the observed value. The value of χ^2 needed for significance at the P = 0.05 level is 3.84, and for P = 0.01, 6.64. We can thus convert the expression to give the values of Φ required at these two levels:

$$\text{Minimum } \Phi = \sqrt{\frac{3.84}{N}} \quad (P = 0.05)$$

$$\text{or } \sqrt{\frac{6.64}{N}} \quad (P = 0.01)$$

Consideration of the minimum Φ needed for significance and the maximum possible Φ for completions that are very easy or very difficult reveals a further limitation of this index: if numbers are sufficiently small, then it becomes mathematically impossible for completions at the extremes of difficulty or easiness to achieve a Φ which differs significantly from zero. Figure 6 shows how the minimum Φ for significance at the 0.05 and 0.01 levels varies with N (plotted on a logarithmic scale). The horizontal dotted lines represent the maximum values of Φ which a question of a given difficulty can yield. We can now see that if the numbers in the examination fall as low as 10, no question with a p of over 0.7 or under 0.3, i.e. one answered correctly by more than 70% or less than 30% of the candidates, can achieve a significant Φ and questions with p outside the limits of 0.4 to 0.6 cannot yield a Φ significant at the 0.01 level. Similarly if questions having p values of 0.1 or 0.9 are to be used, the numbers must not fall below 34 if Φ values significantly different from zero at the 0.05 level are to be obtained; for significance at the 0.01 level at least 60 candidates are required.

Small numbers of candidates and very difficult or very easy questions both tend to reduce the usefulness of any index of discrimination derived from the results; in the case of the Φ coefficient it can be seen that this difficulty takes an unusually acute form.

The tetrachoric correlation coefficient

The last index to be described is the tetrachoric correlation coefficient (r_{tet}). While this is the least reliable of all, because it discards so much information, it is very valuable when the work of computation must be reduced to a minimum - either because no mechanical or electrical aid is available, or because a quick survey to detect gross anomalies, such as those resulting from an ambiguous question or a wrong answer key, is required. Nothing more elaborate than a slide-rule is necessary.

The tetrachoric r should not be used where the possible scores for the question being studied are limited to two values (e.g. +1 and zero): for this situation the Φ coefficient should be used. Ideally both sets of scores (question scores and total examination scores) should be continuous, normally distributed and linearly related; these conditions are reasonably fulfilled, except perhaps that for normal distribution, in, for example, a question of the independent true-false type where the score may range from -5 through zero to +5.

The handling of the total marks is similar to that required for the Φ coefficient: the candidates are arranged in rank order and divided into an upper and a lower half. The scores for the question are now examined. Suppose there are 50 candidates and the distribution of question scores is as follows:

Question score	No. of candidates with this score
-5	0
-4	0
-3	1
-2	0
-1	5
0	8
+1	13
+2	10
+3	9
+4	3
+5	1

The median for this distribution (the value dividing it into two equal parts, such that half the candidates exceed this score and half fall below it) clearly lies somewhere between +1 and +2. Each candidate can now be assigned to one of four categories as shown below:-

	Lower half on question score	Upper half on question score
Upper half on total score	6 (b)	19 (a)
Lower half on total score	21 (d)	4 (c)

By convention the four quarters of the table are labelled a, b, c, d as shown. If we were aiming to calculate the tetrachoric r accurately we would next embark on a long and arduous series of computations. This would quite defeat the purpose of the exercise and so we use an approximation. The value of the expression ad/bc is calculated and the result is entered into the table on page 105 in Appendix B from which an approximate value for the tetrachoric r can be obtained. For the example quoted, ad/bc yields a value of 16.6 which corresponds with a tetrachoric r of +0.81. If bc is greater than ad the resulting (estimated) tetrachoric r must have a negative sign, and is obtained by entering bc/ad into the table.

The significance of an observed value for r_{tet} depends, as in the case of the other indices, on the number of candidates. The problem is discussed in more detail in Appendix B where a simple graphical solution is presented.

Special problems

Questions with three options. Questions of the 'yes/no/don't know' type require special consideration in item analysis. Suppose the correct response to a particular completion is 'False'. The program can be arranged so as to print the numbers or the proportions of candidates responding with 'True' (incorrect response, -1), 'False' (correct response, +1) or making no response at all (zero). Let us imagine the proportions, expressed as percentages, are 30, 60 and 10 respectively.

Decisions of policy now have to be made before item analysis is possible. Firstly, in the matter of 'percent correct': are the 'don't knows' to be regarded as having withdrawn from the question? In that case the percentage will be (60x100) ÷ (60+30) = 66.7. Or do we put the 'don't knows' in the same category as those giving a definite incorrect response? - in which case the percentage of correct answers is 60. Secondly, in the case of discrimination indices the 'don't knows' raise a still more serious problem. If all the information is to be used, it might seem desirable to calculate a Pearson r, with item scores ranging from +1 through zero to -1. However, if we examine the frequency distribution of these scores we have +1, 60 per cent : zero, 10 per cent : -1, 30 per cent. This distribution, which is certainly by no means unusual in practice, is strongly bimodal and it will be recalled that the theoretical conditions for the Pearson r specify two unimodal distributions. Although Pearson r's calculated from data such as we have postulated will give a rough idea of the discrimination, they are not reliable and no conclusions as to significance can safely be drawn. The frequency of responses in the three categories is so variable that the only safe course is to amalgamate two of the categories into one and use indices of correlation suitable for one dichotomized variable, such as the point-biserial r, or the Φ coefficient. Of the three categories, one clearly separates itself from the other two - that of the candidates making the correct response. The other two categories include candidates of varying degrees of ignorance who may reasonably be classed together for the analysis. We can call our two new categories 'right' and 'not right' and this is probably also a sensible dichotomy for determining the percent correct response.

Small numbers of candidates. It may be helpful if, before leaving the subject of discrimination indices, we summarise the problems arising when the number of candidates is small - say 100 or fewer. Numbers of this order are common in class tests and discrimination indices in such tests may be misinterpreted unless the following points are borne in mind:

(a) even with the most reliable of the indices, the Pearson r, substantial changes in the observed value for a question used in identical form on more than one occasion may occur through the operation of chance alone

(b) in the case of the Φ coefficient, the combination of low numbers and a very easy or very difficult question may make the achievement of 'significant' values mathematically impossible

(c) in the case of the tetrachoric correlation coefficient, considerably higher values are needed for a given level of significance than in the case of the other coefficients when the number of candidates is the same

(d) the finding of a discrimination index somewhat below the value needed for significance at the 5 per cent level need not be the signal for the instant discarding of the item responsible. It is worth using the question again unchanged; its future can then be decided in the light of the observed indices in more than one test.

Some suggestions about how to reach a decision in this last situation may be helpful. Provided that two tests yield similar figures for the mean score or the percentage of correct responses for that question, it is possible to combine the discrimination coefficients and test for significance with the higher number of candidates resulting. Combination is simplest in the case of Φ; if the numbers of candidates in the two tests are the same or nearly so, all that is needed is the arithmetical mean of the two Φ coefficients. Combination of two Pearson r's is more complex, but can be achieved graphically by using the figure in Appendix C. Inspection of the figure shows that for values of r of 0.3 and below, the combined r is indistinguishable from the arithmetical mean of the component r's. If either of the component r's is as high as 0.5, some departure from the arithmetical mean may be found, with the combined r being higher than the arithmetical mean.

Combination of two point-biserial r's may be carried out

approximately, by the same technique as is proposed for combining two Pearson r's. No simple technique is available for combining two tetrachoric r's; the only procedure possible is to add the raw data, compute a combined ad/bc and derive the estimated tetrachoric r in the usual way.

RELIABILITY

A proper discussion of this concept as applied to test procedures would involve statistical reasoning of a somewhat abstract kind which would be out of place in this book. We are concerned here with practical procedures which can be applied so as to estimate to what extent our test procedures are, in a technical sense, reliable.

If a test were perfectly reliable then its use on a single occasion would yield a set of candidate scores which would be perfectly reproduced on any subsequent occasion with the same candidates. This is a situation which is seldom explored experimentally, if only because of the obvious fact that administration of the test on the first occasion might substantially affect the candidates' performance on the second occasion. If the interval between the two tests is lengthened to avoid this effect, then other factors - particularly the increasing knowledge and skill of the candidates - will begin to take effect.

Practical tests of reliability therefore are confined to measurements which can be made on the results of a single examination. Here the aim is to see how well the results from part of a test - say half the items - agree with those from the rest. A simple technique is to divide the test into odd and even-numbered items and to treat these halves as two separate tests, comparing the results by calculating Pearson's r from the two sets of scores. (It is of course understood that the whole test will be as nearly as possible homogeneous, testing in a restricted area of knowledge and attributes, with a random distribution of subject matter.) The split-half technique, as it is called, has been criticised because of the arbitrary way in which the division into two halves takes place; other divisions are possible which might yield different results. Consequently more sophisticated methods have been introduced, notably those of Kuder and Richardson, which in effect take into account all possible ways of splitting the test. The formula No.20 published by these authors, and known generally as 'KR20', is the most accurate and widely used, and is discussed in Appendix D.

VALIDITY

In Chapter 2 we have given a brief explanation of the general concept of the validity of a test. As in the case of reliability, full discussion of the mathematical and statistical approach to this concept would be beyond the scope of this book. Suffice it to say that the mathematical treatment applies mainly to predictive validity, and that for this an acceptable 'criterion' is required. The criterion for such an analysis in the case of, for example, a qualifying medical examination would be some measure of how well the candidate, in later years, exhibited the characteristics desirable in a doctor. Formal evaluation of this sort is not available at present and indeed it is hard to see how it could be carried out, considering the great variety of skills and attributes required of doctors practising in different branches of the profession. We may simply note that the mathematical and statistical apparatus exists for assessing the predictive validity of tests; in the absence of suitable criteria it is impossible to apply these methods.

REFERENCES

Fleming, P.R., Manderson, W.G., Matthews, M.B., Sanderson, P.H. and Stokes, J.F. (1974) Evolution of an examination, M.R.C.P. (U.K.). *British Medical Journal*, 1,99.
Guilford, J.P. (1965) *Fundamental Statistics in Psychology and Education*, 4th edition. New York : McGraw - Hill.

8. Organisation of Examinations

The organisation of a large examination in medicine makes great demands on the time of many people, from the examiners to the administrative staff who ensure that candidates are present in the right place at the right time and the medical and nursing staff in whose hands lies much of the responsibility for the efficient running of the clinical examinations - to mention but a few. In recent years the introduction of MCQ and other objective techniques has added a new dimension to the exercise.

There are three aspects to the organisation of any human endeavour - the preliminary planning, the execution of the plan and the review of the results of the exercise; in the succinct jargon of the RAF, briefing, 'op' and debriefing all require attention. We shall, therefore, discuss these three aspects of the organisation of an examination which can be exemplified most clearly in the case of MCQ and other objective question papers.

ORGANISATION OF MCQ PAPERS

The scoring and analysis of MCQ, described in Chapters 6 and 7, generate a large amount of data the handling of which, together with the indexing and storage of the questions, is a task of some complexity. There is much to be said for using the great capacity of a computer for storage and rapid retrieval of information and we shall discuss this matter later. Our own experience, however, has been with a card-index system, with manual retrieval and this account of the organisation of examinations containing MCQ is based on that experience. We do not propose to list the numerous stages in the preparation of a paper from the time the questions are first removed from the bank to the moment, often many months later, when they are replaced. We shall rather emphasise what we believe to be the important principles involved in the process.

MCQs are set by individuals and improved by committees. The larger the source of questions the better and there seems no good reason for confining the construction of questions for an examination to the examiners themselves. (The question of copyright has sometimes been raised. In our view the separate items are no more than the raw material from which papers are constructed and cannot be regarded as subject to copyright. This is not the case, of course, with complete MCQ examination papers of which the copyright is usually held by the examining body concerned.) When a new question is received, it should be scrutinised, either in detail by a test committee (see below) or more cursorily by whoever is responsible for the question bank; this individual we shall refer to, for want of a better name, as the bank manager. We believe that he should be medically qualified and he should be empowered to make minor syntactic amendments to the questions he receives. He should rarely reject a question except when it is exactly or nearly identical to one already in the bank or when it has been submitted in an inappropriate format. Before a question is placed in the bank it should be given a unique index number based on a subject-matter classification. We shall discuss classification and indexing in more detail in connection with computer storage of questions; for a card-index, a fairly simple system is adequate, although scope for a limited amount of cross-referencing is helpful. In an established bank many of the questions will have been used in previous examinations; it is convenient to record, on the cards, details of the previous scoring and item analyses.

When a MCQ paper is to be set, the bank manager selects the required number of questions covering the areas of knowledge to be tested. The proportion of new questions chosen will depend on, among other things, the size of the bank but it is essential that a few questions, perhaps 10 per cent, have been used before in identical form; these are the 'marker' questions (see Chapter 6). Questions which have been used before and have been modified can also be selected but these cannot, of course, function as 'markers'. If all new questions have been scrutinised by a test committee before being placed in the bank, the bank manager could construct the definitive paper. We do not favour this system, however, as questions may become out-of-date as a result of new knowledge with which the bank manager may not be familiar. It is therefore preferable, we believe, to submit the initial selection of questions to a test committee whose responsibility it is to construct the question paper.

The reliability of a MCQ paper depends very largely on the industry and efficiency of the test committee responsible for it. The committee should be large enough to contain specialists in the major areas of knowledge being tested although it should not be so large as to encourage discursive debate. There should probably not be more than about 12 members who should be experienced in the construction of MCQs as well as in their own specialties. There is much to be said for circulating the questions well in advance of the meeting of the committee and for asking each member to be prepared to lead the discussion on a group of questions and to be ready with constructive suggestions for their amendment if necessary. All the members should be provided with the scores and item analyses of questions which have been used before and with the previous versions of questions which have been modified, if only to prevent the same errors of construction being made twice. The work of a test committee is taxing but few find it disagreeable; many members, indeed, have commented that the meetings provide pleasantly informal refresher courses in subjects outside their recent experience.

Little need be said about the final steps in the preparation of the paper, after the meeting of the test committee, except to point out that proof-reading of a MCQ paper must be more than usually careful and that meticulous attention must be paid to the correctness of the answer key. Errors are particularly likely to creep in when a test committee has modified an item and has changed a positive completion to negative or vice versa.

Apart from the construction of the examination paper itself, it is important to ensure that candidates are in no doubt about the method by which they are to record their answers. It is wise to prepare detailed instructions and to send them to candidates well in advance of the examination. In the preparation of these instructions the following points are important:

(a) The format of the questions must be clearly explained; in particular, there must be no confusion in the candidates' minds between five-choice completion questions (in which one completion only can be correct) and independent true-false questions. In this connection, it is worth pointing out that it is unwise to mix several question formats in a single paper unless the candidates are quite familiar with this type of examination

(b) The scoring system must be made clear to the candidates

(c) The method by which candidates are to indicate their choice of completions as true or false (and their examination numbers or other means of identification) must be explained. Great pains must be taken over this explanation especially if, as is usually the case, the answer sheets are to be processed by an automatic document-reader. Candidates must also be told whether they are permitted to alter any of their answers and, if so, how this is to be done.

Automatic document-readers function by detecting either the darkness of the candidates' marks, using an optical system, or the electrical conductivity of marks made with a lead pencil. In the latter case suitable pencils must be provided and candidates must be warned to use only these. It is as well to reiterate these instructions verbally at the time of the examination itself and careful invigilation is necessary to prevent the occasional candidate from adopting his own idiosyncratic method of recording his answers. Fewer problems, naturally, arise in this area if the papers are to be hand-marked or if punch-cards or paper tape, for machine-marking, are to be prepared manually since it is often possible to infer from a doubtful mark what the candidate really intended.

For the marking and analysis of a long MCQ paper with a large number of candidates a computer is almost essential. However, if the paper is fairly short and the number of candidates does not exceed 100 or so, hand-marking is possible, though tedious. No special skills are required and much of the work can be delegated to quite junior staff. Clearly only the simplest marking system can be used, such as +1, 0 or +1, 0, -1 (see Chapter 6) and sophisticated analysis is hardly possible even if a desk calculator is available. A convenient method of hand-marking is described by Lever *et al.*,(1970) and many people have devised similar systems.

A detailed account of computer marking and analysis of MCQs would not be appropriate in this book even if we were competent to give such an account. However, a few general remarks may be helpful to those who propose to introduce computer marking. The first essential is to specify, with great precision, what is required of the computer system. This includes such details as the number of questions, the number of completions within them and the expected number of candidates. In addition, naturally, the computer scientists must be told whether scoring of the answers alone is required or whether the candidates are to be ranked as well; also the nature of the item-analysis must be specified. Scoring per se is a relatively simple exercise and can be performed on quite a small desk computer. However, once it becomes necessary to store candidates' scores for ranking or item analysis, the size of the computer becomes critical. The array of data is a function of the number of candidates and the number of completions and the larger this product the larger must be the storage capacity of the computer in terms of core size and number of discs available; tape storage is feasible but adds considerably to the time of running the program. The preparation of a suitable program will take a skilled programmer about a month; the actual writing of the program is less time-consuming than the checking as each step in the prototype program has to be checked by manual calculation. Once the program is written the actual scoring and analysis of an examination paper is very rapid; however, if a document-reader is not available, time must be allowed for the punching and verification of cards; for a paper of 60 independent true-false questions taken by 70 candidates this takes one person about 8 hours. Finally, it is unwise to ask for any modification of the program, however trivial it may seem, without allowing ample time. Once a program has been modified, it has to be checked in toto once again. There is no need for examiners to acquire any expertise in computer science but, as often in professional life, a nodding acquaintance with the problems of ones colleagues goes a long way to ensure amicable and fruitful collaboration.

After the examination is over, the extent to which the predetermined objectives have been achieved must be investigated. It is customary to hold a final meeting of examiners to decide on the pass-mark and on such matters as the award of honours. We believe that much more is required and that a detailed review of all the questions together with the analysis is most important. This review should be undertaken by a test committee, preferably the same as the one which set the paper, who should be provided with all the relevant data on the questions. As before, individual members should be invited to comment on groups of questions and to suggest modifications in the light of the analysis. Only in this way, we believe, can members of test committees acquire the expertise necessary for the construction of good MCQs. If, as we have suggested, the original questions were acquired from many sources, it will rarely be possible to involve all the authors personally in the detailed review. It is, however, courteous to provide those who have taken the trouble to construct MCQs with some information on how their questions have performed in an examination. Most people seem to welcome this information and find it helps them when next they undertake the construction of MCQs. In some cases it is also desirable to give the candidates details of their performance (see Chapter 9).

Computer storage of MCQs

As we have said, our experience in this area is limited but it seems such a logical stage in the development of a MCQ bank that some comments, however theoretical, are necessary.
There would seem to be little difficulty in the storage of the text of all versions of the questions, together with details of the candidates' scores and the indices of discrimination; a record of the previous occasions on which a question was used and, possibly, of its source, would also be required. Unused questions could also be stored, perhaps after scrutiny, and modification if necessary, by a test committee. Careful thought would need to be given to the classification of the questions so that it would be possible to instruct the computer to select material for an examination paper with the appropriate balance between the various areas of knowledge being tested, with specified numbers of new and used questions and, in the case of the latter, of an appropriate order of difficulty. There should also be provision for the selection of the required number of marker questions. Another important requirement would be that overlap between different questions should be avoided and here problems of classification might well arise. Unless each question were classified under a main subject heading with, in addition, cross references to all the topics covered in the several completions, overlapping and even duplication of topics might occur in a single paper. For example, in a question on the causes of hypercalcaemia, sarcoidosis might well appear as a positive completion; in a question selected from a different section of the bank, with the stem 'Recognised features of sarcoidosis include', hypercalcaemia might well be one of the completions. Without extensive cross-referencing, it would be possible to ask the same question twice over in the same paper. If these problems could be overcome, as presumably they could, a computer might well become as indispensable to the manager of

a MCQ bank as it is, we understand, to his financial counterpart.

The preparation of an examination paper by a computer would require some means of display of the questions. Probably a visual display unit of some kind would be appropriate for initial inspection but it would be necessary for the system to provide hard copies of the selected questions. These, which should include all the relevant statistical information would be needed by the test committee who could not be superseded by the computer. Automatic pre-selection of a batch of appropriate questions is certainly feasible and, probably, acceptable but we do not believe that the time has yet come when the construction of a definitive examination paper can be safely left to a computer.

OTHER OBJECTIVE TECHNIQUES

The organisation of examinations containing the type of short open-ended questions which we have discussed in Chapter 3 presents similar problems to that of MCQ papers. The work of the test committees includes not only attention to the wording of the questions, a particularly difficult task when a long case-history has to be edited, but also prediction of all the likely answers and allocation of appropriate scores; in addition, arrangements must be made for hand-scoring of the answers by adequately briefed examiners. Review of the papers after the examination in the light of the statistical analysis is as important as with MCQs. Additional problems arise if pattern recognition is to be tested by confronting the candidates with Xrays, colour photographs, ECGs and the like. A decision has to be made as to whether this material is to be reproduced in the examination paper or presented in some other way. Black and white material, such as ECGs, can be reproduced quite easily and accurately but, although some examining bodies are using colour photographs and reproductions of Xrays in their examination papers, we are, at present, not completely satisfied with the quality of reproduction which can be achieved without inordinate expense. In our opinion, coloured photographs are better presented as transparencies and, as it is hardly feasible to provide each candidate with his own set of slides, projection of the material has to be arranged. Much the same applies to X-rays although we accept that, even in the best transparencies, much fine detail is lost and we know of no completely satisfactory method of presenting Xrays to large numbers of candidates at, or about, the same time.

If projected material is to be used, care must be taken to ensure that all candidates have an equally satisfactory view of the screen; some details of the type of projection facilities required are given in Appendix E (we are indebted to Dr. Peter Hansell for this information). If an examination is being taken in several centres simultaneously it also becomes necessary to arrange that viewing conditions are, as nearly as possible, identical in all the centres. Our experience with projected material has convinced us that this is a feasible method of testing certain attributes but there is no doubt that, if it becomes possible to reproduce, on paper, all the required material faithfully and cheaply, this would be preferable.

OTHER TYPES OF EXAMINATION

Most examining bodies have great experience in the organisation of written examinations and of orals, practicals and clinicals and it would be presumptuous of us to attempt a detailed account of the procedures involved. Perhaps, however, we may be permitted to make a few points which do not always receive the attention they deserve.

We have already suggested, in Chapters 3 and 4, various ways in which these parts of an examination may be improved and it follows, as a corollary of these suggestions, that more time than is usually allowed for the preliminary examiners' meeting is required to permit full discussion and agreement on the attributes to be tested in the various parts of the examination and on the details of the marking system which is to be used.

The venue of clinical examinations is another topic which, we think, deserves a little discussion. This is usually a ward or wards of one, or more often several, hospitals but, in some examinations, a large hall is used. On the whole we prefer the former arrangement because it seems intrinsically more appropriate to ask candidates to examine patients in their, temporary, natural habitat; it is thus possible to include a wider variety of cases in the examination, among them patients whom one would be reluctant to transport to an examination hall. Against this must be set the fact that a hospital-based examination is uneconomical of professional manpower, requiring, as it does, the nearly full-time services of a registrar or other assistant while the examination is in progress. In an examination hall fewer assistants are required in relation to the number of candidates being examined. Furthermore, there is something to be said for a system in which all the examiners meet regularly and have an opportunity to discuss the cases being used. It is our impression that it is easier to keep the standard of a clinical examination constant in these circumstances than when the examiners work in pairs, or quartets, in a hospital and only meet their colleagues from other hospitals at a final examiners' meeting, if then.

A CENTRAL MEDICAL EXAMINATIONS SERVICE

In 1968 the Royal Commission on Medical Education stated, in connection with the need for reform of examinations, 'We think an appropriate organisation.....should be charged with the responsibility of studying (methods of assessment) and, perhaps, of providing a service to universities and post-graduate training bodies on the lines of that offered in the United States of America by the National Board of Medical Examiners'. In consequence of this the Association for the Study of Medical Education (ASME) convened a meeting in 1969 to determine what support there might be for such an organisation. There was initially a very encouraging response and a Working Party was set up which reported to a second ASME meeting two years later. By this time very much less support was forthcoming and the proposal that such an organisation, which was to have been called the Central Medical Examinations Service (CMES), should be set up, was shelved. Because we believe that such an organisation could play an important role in medical education in this country, we think that it would be appropriate for us to re-examine some of the proposals of that Working Party of which we were members.

Two main functions were envisaged for CMES - service and research. The estimate of the service need was based on the view that 'a considerable increase in the total quantity of testing could be expected'. (Quotations in this section are from the report of the Working Party,1971). This view has since been amply confirmed with a further increase in the numbers of medical students, a greater use of in-course assessment, the institution of new postgraduate examinations and an increase in the number of candidates entering for long-established examinations. In view of the considerable burden imposed by examinations on the staff of medical schools and of postgraduate organisations it was considered that 'the primary service role of any central unit must be to relieve individual teachers, departments, schools and postgraduate authorities of as much of the technical burden of examining as possible, without any interference with their responsibilities'. We now suspect that this role may be an impossible one for CMES to fill and will discuss this matter further below.

The proposals for research to be carried out by CMES were, we believe, not contentious and included projects, to be carried out in collaboration with medical schools and other organisations, on improving the quality of written, oral and practical examinations.

The importance of CMES being completely independent of all other educational and examining bodies was emphasised in the report of the Working Party and it was stated that 'it is of great importance that CMES does not attempt or appear to attempt to establish pass-marks or in any way to usurp the functions of any examining body.' It was envisaged that the test committees set up by CMES would construct MCQs and assemble them into examination papers which would be taken, in part or as a whole, by candidates in many medical schools. The papers would be scored and analysed by CMES and the results, including comparative data if desired, transmitted to the schools concerned.

We now feel somewhat uneasy with the concept of a test committee setting an examination paper without any idea of the educational objectives of individual schools. It may be that this dilemma was one of the reasons why the Working Party's proposals were shelved, rather than the considerable financial implications which seemed, at the time, to be an important factor. Having emphasised, as we have done, that examinations are, or ought to be, an integral part of the educational process, it would be somewhat inconsistent if we were to suggest that an examination, set by a committee outside the teaching faculties, would be suitable *as a part of the courses* of all those faculties.

We remain convinced of the need for some form of central organisation if only to avoid unnecessary duplication of efforts, in many centres, in this area. We are now less certain about the service role of such an organisation and it may be that, as the Royal Commission originally hinted, the initial responsibility of a central examinations service should be for research. One of the first, and most important, research projects could be an attempt to determine the best way of providing a service to autonomous examining bodies.

REFERENCES

Lever, R.S., Harden, R.M., Wilson, G.M. and Jolley, J.L. (1970) A simple answer sheet designed for use with objective examinations. *British Journal of Medical Education*, 4, 37.

Report of a working party on a central medical examinations service (1971) London : Association for the Study of Medical Education.

Royal Commission on Medical Education (1968) *Report*, Cmnd 3569. London : H.M.S.O.

9. Progressive Assessment

We have already, in Chapter 5, expressed our opinion that the assessment of attitudes is more likely to be reliable and acceptable to teachers and students if it is carried out progressively throughout the course of training. It remains to discuss what role in-course assessment can, or should, play in examinations in the cognitive and psychomotor domains.

In any course of training, particularly the undergraduate course, it is common practice to incorporate assessment of one form or another. This ranges from verbal questioning during tutorials to formal examination at various stages; it also commonly includes reports from teachers in the various departments through which the student passes. Thus a good deal of information of varying quality is accumulated which can be used to monitor a student's progress and to provide the teachers with feedback on the efficacy of their teaching. Few would disagree that in-course, or progressive, assessment is of considerable value in this respect. However, it is when it is used as a partial or total replacement for the final examination that there is considerable difference of opinion and, before proceeding to a discussion of the methods of in-course assessment, it seems reasonable to review the arguments for and against its use in this way.

Protagonists of the traditional final examination maintain that it is important to encourage students to review and consolidate their knowledge at the end of the course. Although this is true, such an argument is tantamount to an admission that the examination itself is of secondary importance in comparison with the period of revision preceding it. Another argument which has been advanced is that it is as important to assess the finished product of an educational process as it is to test an article coming off the end of a production line. Continuing this not wholly appropriate industrial analogy it can be argued that the final inspection need be no more than cursory provided that the earlier stages of the process have been carefully monitored.

Those who favour progressive assessment have emphasised the stress induced by final examinations in which the knowledge and skills acquired over the years are assessed in a few critical hours. Few candidates face examinations with complete equanimity and, for some, 'examination nerves' can be a serious problem. If it were certain that this stress could be reduced by progressive assessment, this would be a powerful argument in its favour.

However, each item in a programme of progressive assessment contributes its own quota of stress and this may cause chronic anxiety which is as serious as the acute anxiety induced by finals. A particular problem arises with the 'slow starter', the student who finds considerable difficulty in the early months of a course and may feel that he is falling so far behind his colleagues as to make ultimate failure inevitable. As Miller and Parlett (1974) have said: 'There may well be a type of Parkinson's Law operating: that stress and examination preparation increase to fill the space and time available'.

A final point concerns the role of examinations as an aid to forgetting. Miller and Parlett (1974) quote the views of the Chairman of the Department of Psychology at the Massachusetts Institute of Technology on this 'memory-clearing' function of examinations. This concept that an examination is seen as a terminal task which, when completed, 'wipes the slate clean' is supported by psychological studies of memory which have shown that the retention of a half-completed problem is better than that of one which has been wholly completed. Certainly many clinical teachers are familiar with the ignorance displayed by junior clinical students of subjects such as anatomy in which they have recently been examined. This aspect of examinations is relevant to a discussion on progressive assessment in several ways. On the one hand it may be argued that, if a subject such as obstetrics is wholly taught and examined early in the undergraduate course, it will be forgotten well before the end of that course. On the other hand, even if this subject were incorporated in a final examination, it seems probable that it would thereafter be forgotten anyway and deferment of amnesia for a year or so seems a rather modest educational objective. If students can be persuaded that each item of progressive assessment is to be regarded as a test of, as yet, incomplete knowledge, this knowledge, by virtue of the fact that it is incomplete, should be retained more readily. Retention will be all the more likely if it is clear that knowledge acquired and tested early in the course will be applied in the later years. Experience suggests, however, that this may not be as simple as it sounds as students have their own, often inaccurate, ideas about what is or is not relevant; however, recognition of this problem goes some way towards its solution. The reduction in size and importance of the final examination can be expected to prevent wholesale memory clearance once the undergraduate course is over, especially if 'finals' is seen merely as one more item in progressive assessment leading to a pre-registration period which is recognised by all concerned as part of the whole educational process. On balance, we are of the opinion that progressive assessment should replace much of the traditional undergraduate examination system and we believe that most of its alleged disadvantages can be obviated by designing a flexible system which combines both the monitoring and examining components.

The application of progressive assessment to the postgraduate field is more difficult but it should be feasible if the appropriate course of training leading to an examination has been defined in detail.

We would have liked to suggest, in support of our contention, that the dismantling of the traditional final examination would lead to a saving of time and money; it is, however, unlikely that progressive assessment, if it is carried out properly, would be any simpler or cheaper to organise. The arguments in its favour, which we shall develop further below, are academic not economic.

THE APPLICATION OF PROGRESSIVE ASSESSMENT

Hitherto, in this chapter, we have referred to in-course assessment and progressive assessment as if they were synonymous. We suggest that this is not the case and that, although a series of weekly, monthly or quarterly examinations can be correctly regarded as in-course assessment, such a programme does not justify the use of the term 'progressive' unless the knowledge and skills assessed have been acquired in a logical sequence. For this reason, it seems to us that progressive assessment can be usefully discussed only in relation to the design of an undergraduate curriculum or of a postgraduate course of training. We propose therefore to outline some of the principles which should influence the planning of a medical course, with particular reference to progressive assessment.

The development of academic preclinical and clinical departments and the increasing specialisation of modern medicine, which are admirably adapted to the advancement of knowledge and to the provision of efficient medical care, have resulted in the undergraduate medical course becoming more and more subject-centred. Thus, in many clinical schools, a student passes from one special department to another, acquiring knowledge and skills in small packets each of which can be separately assessed. The sum-total of such in-course assessments could be regarded as equal to a final examination but such a system incorporates the disadvantage of recurrent memory clearance to which we have referred. Some of the inter-departmental barriers have been broken down by integrated teaching but the fact remains that much medical teaching is still subject-centred rather than student-centred.

It occurs to us that it might be more profitable to recognise that students begin their studies of medicine, or of any other subject, by acquiring facts which they later learn to relate to each other; later still these relationships are made use of in the appreciation of a total situation and in the solution of problems. Such a taxonomical approach, which has been discussed in Chapter 2, would permit assessment to be more truly progressive in that, in the early part of a course, a student's knowledge and understanding of facts could be assessed;

only later would he be tested on more sophisticated matters such as the interpretation of data and the solution of problems. Likewise, in the psychomotor domain, particularly in the clinical disciplines, it would be reasonable, early in the course, to test a student's ability to elicit physical signs more or less in isolation and only later to require him to analyse his findings, using his recently acquired problem-solving ability, to produce a diagnosis. Some medical schools have already taken a step in this direction by arranging for the majority, or all, of the written papers to be taken before the end of the course and for the final examination to be entirely clinical in which the higher taxonomic attributes of the cognitive and psychomotor domains can be assessed. Clearly a curriculum in which the early months were devoted exclusively to the acquisition of facts in all the medical disciplines would be administratively unworkable. However, we believe that some change of emphasis in this direction, permitting assessment along the lines we have indicated, would be salutary.

Many of the techniques which can be used in progressive assessment have already been discussed and require brief comment only. For example, multiple-choice questions are very suitable for testing in the lower taxonomic levels of the cognitive domain - knowledge and understanding of facts - and could be used freely in the early part of a course. Later, more use could be made of open-ended questions involving data-interpretation and problem-solving such as have been described in Chapter 3. In the psychomotor domain, manual dexterity in practical work and skill in the elicitation of physical signs could be assessed first; here, check-lists of the required skills, discussed in Chapter 4, would be appropriate. In practice clinical assessment could be quite informal at this stage, being carried out, en passant, by the student's own teachers. In the final year, the student's ability to deal with a clinical problem could be assessed, perhaps by means of 'long cases' in a traditional clinical examination. Alternatively, or in addition, this is an area in which use might well be made of Problem-Oriented Medical Records - POMR (Weed, 1969). Apart from the undoubted value of POMR in improving medical care, it seems to be a very useful tool in the assessment of a student's depth of understanding of a clinical situation. The POMR system, with its rigorous insistence on the sequence - observation : inference : action - reveals errors of reasoning with startling clarity and we believe that it should be used much more widely both in teaching and in assessment.

A source of information which, perhaps with some adaptation, could lend itself well to progressive assessment is a series of reports on a student's progress made by the teachers in the departments and clinical firms through which he passes. The reliability of this commonly-used system as an assessment technique depends critically on the format in which the reports are made. In this connection, many of the points on design of questionnaires, made in Chapter 5, are relevant: Miller (1961) also has a useful chapter on this topic. The views of the teachers on a student's knowledge, skills and attitudes can be sought by appropriate questions and a simple scaling system should be devised for the recording of their answers. Complexity should be avoided as teachers are busy and students numerous. Another point worth bearing in mind is that the propensity to choose the modal point on a scale is as common among teachers as among students and, as pointed out in Chapter 5, a scale with an even number of points (usually four) is desirable for this reason.

Consideration must next be given to the problem of those students whose performance in the early stages of a programme of progressive assessment is unsatisfactory. It is very difficult to distinguish the slow starters from those who should never have started. It is here, of course, that the monitoring role of progressive assessment becomes important so that a single failure becomes no more than an indication that more time is needed by that particular student to complete that part of the course. In the long run this may mean that some will require longer than the statutory number of years to reach graduation. We hope that this fact will become more widely appreciated, particularly by local education authorities. Students who fail repeatedly at an early stage present a particular problem and it may well be kindest, in the long run, to advise some of them to give up their plans for a medical career. It may be possible, however, to identify some who, while failing on more than one occasion to reach the pass mark, have nevertheless improved significantly and an arbitrary rejection after a specified number of failures cannot always be justified. At the other end of the spectrum of ability, there seems no good reason, other than administrative convenience, why the ablest students should not present themselves for an item of progressive assessment earlier than the majority of their colleagues. Such students - most of them likely to become honours graduates - could then be allowed, indeed encouraged, to use the time they have saved in extensive elective studies from which they will, by virtue of their ability, be able to profit more than most.

Apart from all the other advantages of progressive assessment which we have discussed, it seems to us that the most important benefit accruing from its use is the ability to cater for students of all degrees of competence without either undue pressure on the weak or tedium for the best. Karl Marx's aphorism, slightly mis-quoted, 'To each according to his abilities, to each according to his needs' is surely applicable even in a capitalist educational system.

REFERENCES

Miller, G.E. (1961), ed. *Teaching and learning in medical school.*

Cambridge, Mass: Harvard University Press.
Miller, C.M.L. and Parlett, M. (1974) *Up to the mark: a study of the examination game*. London: Society for Research into Higher Education.
Weed, L.L. (1969) *Medical Records, Medical Education, and Patient Care*. Chicago: Year Book Medical Publishers.

10. A Look to the Future

Though speculation is no substitute for hard work, we feel able, as we approach the end of this book, to think aloud about some of the major problems which remain in the field of evaluation.

THE GRADUATING EXAMINATION

It seems probable that the importance of the 'final' examination will diminish in the face of increased use by schools of progressive assessment as set out in Chapter 9.

The principle of institutional responsibility, which allows each school to experiment with its own educational ideas and priorities, is already generally accepted within the traditional framework. If this trend continues, wider variations between schools are bound to occur and problems may arise in ensuring uniformity of standard. The situation could arise where students from Optimborough might pick up the best jobs in later life, those from Middleton the humdrum, while the graduates of Lower Scoring might find themselves at a serious disadvantage.

This state of affairs might be prevented by arranging for the students of all schools to sit a common examination at the time of graduation, perhaps under the aegis of a reconstituted General Medical Council, which, at the same time, could provide the extra-mural challenge, the need for which is likely to be felt by some students.

If a common examination, such as that offered by the National Board of Medical Examiners in Philadelphia, became desirable, it would have to cover a wide area of knowledge and might occupy the inside of a day; this would need to be the same day at each school, but the arrangement of this would not present a serious problem; the main part of a school's graduating examination (even if it were not fragmented throughout the course) could take place at any time and the use made (if any) of the common test in the graduation decision remain entirely a matter for the individual school. Under these circumstances, the need for some sort of central organisation such as has been outlined in Chapter 8, will be apparent.

COMPUTER-BASED EXAMINATIONS

In the meanwhile, much work is being carried out in North America in polishing, refining and gaining experience in the computer-based examination (CBX) and it seems likely that this approach to evaluation may in time take root (Senior 1973). CBX certainly provides a realistic exercise in problem-solving and decision-taking. It has already been shown that patients in Britain talk quite comfortably to a computer (some patients feel more at ease with it than they do with the doctor) and there is no reason to suppose that medical students will react in a different way. The main limiting factors in its general use at present are expense, the small number of problem-solving programs currently available and the difficulties of scoring.

The first two of these may become less important with the passage of time and the ease of resolution of the third will depend partly on which type of CBX is finally chosen, the 'index' or the 'free response' form. Either type of CBX operates effectively as an educational training instrument (answers to questions can be built into the program so as to steer students away from unprofitable lines of enquiry), showing the diagnostic paths and therapeutic approaches used by the student; the complexities of scoring a 'free response' test are considerable and the program itself has, of course, to be much more elaborate in order to cover all anticipated eventualities. This may limit its value as a test instrument.

CONTINUING EDUCATION

The speed of expansion of the technological aspects of a doctor's knowledge have led not only to increased specialisation but also to an instinctive wish by many doctors for some sort of re-integrative process, so as to be able to understand at least the broad lines along which specialties other than their own are developing. Self-assessment programmes, so ably pioneered by the American College of Physicians and already offered by fourteen specialty boards in the USA, amplify and formalise this approach. Perhaps more important, every ward round and every clinical conference provides a medical audit situation at which we are judged, even if silently, by our colleagues, though the criteria of effective performance are not clearly defined and the educational message will only reach those who are prepared to receive it.

In the USA the opportunities for taking part in continuing medical education are enormous. About two thirds of all practising physicians sign up for one course a year; this is, of course, no guarantee that they attend all of it, or if they do, that they stay awake, or, if they do not sleep, that they derive any benefit from the experience. Such courses are sometimes designed in too narrow terms without sufficient prior identification of patient care needs and incorporate a mass of factual data with little in the way of problem-solving.

These courses are used by some American states (Kansas, Kentucky, Maryland and New Mexico, so far) as a sort of relicensure test; certified evidence of about 150 hours of continuing medical education in three years is required from any doctor who wishes to continue practising medicine in these states. Such evidence may also earn him a Physicians Recognition Award which affords him some financial benefit in that he has to pay a less high premium for insurance against a 'malpractice' claim.

Such evidence as is available does not suggest any close relationship between regularity of attendance at continuing medical education sessions and the quality of medical care delivered. The latter needs to be assessed by observation of a man at his daily work, in familiar surroundings, that is at a medical audit. We believe that, if it is considered desirable in Britain to undertake some ongoing re-evaluation of a man's competence to continue independent medical practice, this is the tool which might most reasonably be used; it would be best carried out at a local level by trusted colleagues and the loss of objectivity that this approach implies would be more than compensated for by the absence of the tensions which would inevitably be engendered by a central team of assessors. Guide lines for local teams could, of course, be prepared by national or regional bodies and much thought would need to be given to the standards of performance expected. This is one of the problems which must now be exercising those in the USA who will be responsible for the application of the Professional Standards Review Organisation Law, due to come into operation in 1976.

Relicensure and recertification

These American terms may be unfamiliar to English readers. Licensure is equivalent to full registration in Britain; certification implies the possession of a specialist postgraduate diploma.

The concept of hiring a diploma rather than having it for life is becoming widespread in the United States and, though the demands for relicensure have not yet been clearly defined, the question of recertification at the postgraduate level has received rather more detailed attention, partly as a result of pressure from commercial insurance carriers who pay such a high proportion of the cost of illness.

The American Board of Medical Specialties has recommended the concept of periodic re-examination to its component specialty boards. The American Board of Internal Medicine (ABIM) has already offered a voluntary recertification examination and this may become compulsory in a few years time. Large numbers will be involved and the examination can only take the form of a written test as it does at present and must ignore the clinical skills at the bedside and the attitudes which contribute so much to the effectiveness of an experienced doctor. At present the responsibility for declaring that an ABIM candidate is adequately equipped in this sense is delegated to the physician in charge of his training course, but for the recertification of a man established in independent practice no such assessment will be available.

The challenge facing those who might be entrusted with the onerous task of organising some sort of recertification procedure in Britain would be to give adequate weight to the qualities of reliability, initiative, integrity, resilience and capacity for sensible choice which all agree they would like to see in our doctors, but which cannot be measured with any great confidence at present.

THE COMMON MARKET

Any country that is a member of the European Economic Community has to face the problem raised by free movement of doctors to practise in countries other than those in which they trained.

It is common knowledge that courses of undergraduate training (and, possibly, their objectives) vary quite widely between individual countries of 'the nine' (Charvat *et al*, 1968). It is probably true to say that British students are more intensively exposed to patients at the bedside than their counterparts in some other European countries, who are expected to absorb their medical education through the more passive medium of the didactic lecture. This is at least partly due to the comparatively large numbers in training. In some countries no-one who elects to embark on a career in medicine is refused a place at medical school, though there is a heavy fall-out in the early years of training. One consequence of this policy may be that these countries have been able to undertake the health care of their nationals with only very little assistance from outside, unlike Britain whose health services are so heavily dependent on expatriate help.

One reason why expatriate doctors who come to Britain for postgraduate training elect to stay on in a career post is that they have some facility with the English language. Lack of this facility in some continental doctors is likely to limit their movement from the rest of the EEC into Britain, quite apart from the fall in earnings such a move would involve. The British are not notable linguists and may well stay at home, despite the financial attractions of practice on the European mainland; it is possible, however, that there may be some movement among those disciplines, such as anaesthetics and radiology, which it is possible to practise within the confines of a limited vocabulary. As countries such as Canada become self-sufficient in terms of medical manpower, Europe may command more attention from those dissatisfied with professional life in Britain.

If, in the future, any restrictions were to be placed on the present free movement within the Community, the need might arise for some sort of test of competence to practise. In this case the effect of translation of test material from one language to another would need careful study. The problems might not be of quite the same order as those, for instance, in Thailand, where examinations are set in the Thai language and script, liberally peppered with English words and phrases for which there is no Thai equivalent, but such evidence as is available suggests that the nuances of communication may become blurred in the course of translation and that different cultural backgrounds may lead to different interpretations of the same question.

In the province of Quebec examinations are set in French as well as English; this has demanded some effort and, though it has achieved a great measure of success, it is understood that French-speaking candidates like to have a sight of the English version of the test paper. The 'tripod' experiment in which an attempt was made to compare standards at one English, one French and one German-speaking school ran into substantial linguistic difficulties.

Movement in the direction of a common test would be easier if the EEC were to adopt a common language, but, as Sampson (1968) reminds us, international languages have not gained wide acceptance - there are only eight million speakers of Esperanto and other tongues such as Volapük and Idiom Neutral are well behind. It would be arrogant to suggest that lingua Britannica may become the lingua franca of international evaluation, but it is probably true that anglophones have at their disposal greater expertise in this field than others. A recent international working party convened under the auspices of the Ciba Foundation has shown that there are good possibilities for the exchange of test material in medicine between English-speaking countries.

THE ECFMG AND TRAB EXAMINATIONS

For many years the United States has sought to ensure a minimum level of competence in those doctors who wish to practise in the country without an American degree by means of a screening examination provided by the Educational Council for Foreign Medical Graduates (ECFMG). This consists of two parts, one a test of ability to understand English language and the other a MCQ assessment of factual information.

There has been a great deal of dissatisfaction in the USA, however, with the limited scope of the ECFMG Examination to the point that a certain cynicism has emerged among employing authorities which has resulted in the appearance of a 'medical underground' of FMGs who have not passed the ECFMG test and who are working nevertheless in various capacities in the health field, outside the approved training programmes. A recent publication by the National Board of Medical Examiners (1973) takes the view that 'at the present time there is no policy that regulates effectively the immigration of foreign physicians'.

The Temporary Registration Assessment Board (TRAB) set up by the General Medical Council to take stock of foreign graduates from schools which have ceased to enjoy traditional reciprocal arrangements for practice with Britain (British Medical Journal, 1974), has, since June 1975, provided an examination which superficially resembles the ECFMG test with the addition of a modified essay question and an oral test at which candidate and examiner meet face to face. At present TRAB has not found itself able to provide any assessment of clinical method or of capacity to relate to patients and deliver medical care effectively. We think that the absence of such assessment is probably one of the main reasons why the ECFMG has been so heavily criticised, and we hope that TRAB will be able to offer a more comprehensive test in time, as implied in Section 194 of the Merrison report (1975). We believe that a properly organised clinical attachment scheme would provide the best answer to this problem. The dangers of creating a two-tier system of medical care are clearly illustrated by American experience.

THE SO-CALLED DEVELOPING COUNTRIES

Despite the obvious advantages of international movement in terms of exchange of ideas and improved communication between countries, there must be some moral worry about the encouragement of so many nationals from India, Pakistan, Bangladesh, Sri Lanka and elsewhere to contribute to health services in Britain in the face of the pressing needs of patients in their home countries, especially in the rural areas. This is a problem, however, which cannot be answered satisfactorily by any action taken by Britain alone. There is a tendency in these countries to give emphasis in training to a Westernised type of medicine which is still considered highly prestigious in their urban areas. Some of their doctors find opportunities to practise Western medicine in their home country; others finding themselves ill-equipped for work in the rural communities and perhaps reluctant to practise a type of medicine they have seen undervalued in the course of their training, turn their backs on their country of origin and seek a more sophisticated niche overseas. Until these countries take a radical look at the objectives of the medical education they provide, their rural areas will remain underprivileged from the point of view of health care and there will continue to be a steady stream of other people's doctors knocking on Britain's door. We should give these countries all the help we can in developing their postgraduate education and evaluation. In such disciplines as obstetrics and gynaecology and surgery, we can train their doctors in techniques which will be locally useful; obstructed labour is much the same all over the world. In medicine, our help can only be wholly effective if there is a local will to pay greater attention to the problem of nutritional anaemia in the rural areas than to that of supra-sellar cysts in the city.

COST EFFECTIVENESS

We believe that this important subject should receive more attention in the future and that evaluation procedures should take account of probability theory and cost effectiveness (Card and Good, 1971; Card, 1973). That is to say, we should take some account of the probable value of a piece of information in relation to its cost to the patient in terms of discomfort, to the doctor in terms of time and to the state in terms of money.

Not much is known about this yet but such studies as have been made suggest that much of the information we collect in the course of history taking and physical examination is irrelevant and redundant. And, as Cochrane (1972) remarks 'what one needs here is a measurement of the probability of improved outcome for the patients as each new test is added to the repertoire, together with the cost of each test and its risks'.

CONCLUSION

From what has been said, it seems likely that the overall need for evaluation will remain and probably expand in the more difficult areas. Much care and effort will be called for if we are to ensure that our tests are reliable and, even more important, that they are valid for the purposes for which they are designed.

REFERENCES

Card, W.I. (1973) The computing approach to clinical diagnosis. *Proceedings of the Royal Society B,* 184, 421.
Card, W.I. and Good, I.J. (1971) Logical foundations of medicine. *British Medical Journal,* 1, 718.
Charvat, J., McGuire, C. and Parsons, V. (1968) *A Review of the Nature and Uses of Examinations in Medical Education.* Geneva : World Health Organisation.
Cochrane, A.L. (1972) *Effectiveness and Efficiency.* London : The Nuffield Provincial Hospitals Trust.
Committee of Inquiry into the Regulation of the Medical Profession. (1975). *Report,* Cmnd. 6018. London : H.M.S.O.
Leading article (1974) Proposed tests for overseas doctors. *British Medical Journal,* 2, 606.
National Board of Medical Examiners. (1973) *Evaluation in the continuum of medical education.* Philadelphia : National Board of Medical Examiners.
Sampson, A. (1968) *The New Europeans.* London : Hodder and Stoughton.
Senior, J.R. (1973) *Progress in computer-based evaluation in competence.* Philadelphia : American Board of Internal Medicine.

Appendix A:
Significance of Correlation Coefficients for Varying Numbers of Observations

Values of r are read off along the vertical scale in Figure 7. The horizontal scale represents log t, where t is calculated from the equation

$$t = \frac{r\sqrt{N-2}}{\sqrt{1-r^2}}$$

The curved lines connect the relevant points for a selected series of numbers of observations. The dotted lines connect the points on these curves at which P = 0.05 and P = 0.01.

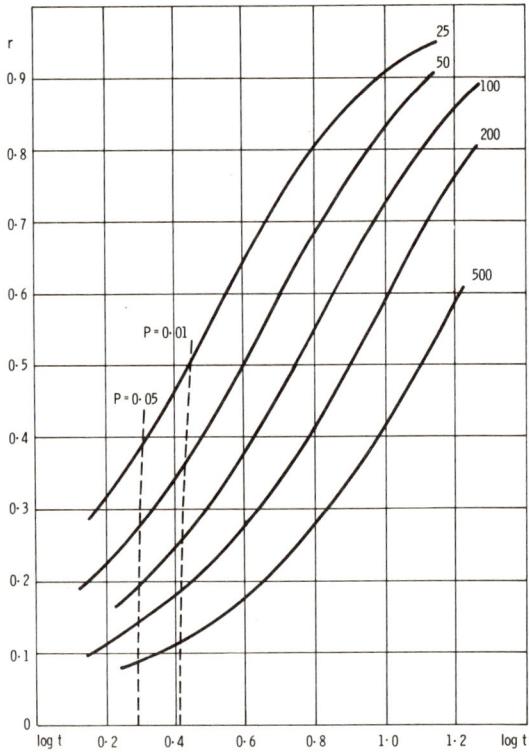

Fig. 7.   *Relationship between product-moment correlation coefficient and log t for varying numbers of observations (see text for details).*

To find the correlation coefficient for a particular number of observations which would have the same significance as an observed coefficient for a greater or less number of observations, proceed as follows. Find a curve which corresponds nearly with the number of observations from which the reference coefficient is derived. Using interpolation between curves if necessary, find the value of log t which corresponds with the observed correlation coefficient. Now refer to a curve which corresponds as nearly as possible with the number of observations for the new coefficient, and read off the value of r corresponding to the value of log t previously found.

Suppose we have as our standard of comparison a value for r of 0.30 for 500 observations (or candidates). We wish to know what value r should reach to have equivalent significance when there are only 100 candidates. From r = 0.30 the curve for N = 500 gives us a value for log t of about 0.85. If this figure is now transferred to the curve for N = 100 we see that a value for r of 0.58 is required for the smaller number of candidates.

This procedure ignores the fact that the value of t (and hence of log t) corresponding to a given level of probability varies slightly with N, but it provides a useful rough guide as to significance levels.

Appendix B:
Determination and Significance of a Tetrachoric Correlation Coefficient

Calculation of the standard error of a tetrachoric r is laborious and we therefore restrict our enquiries about an observed r_{tet} to one point only: does it differ significantly from zero?

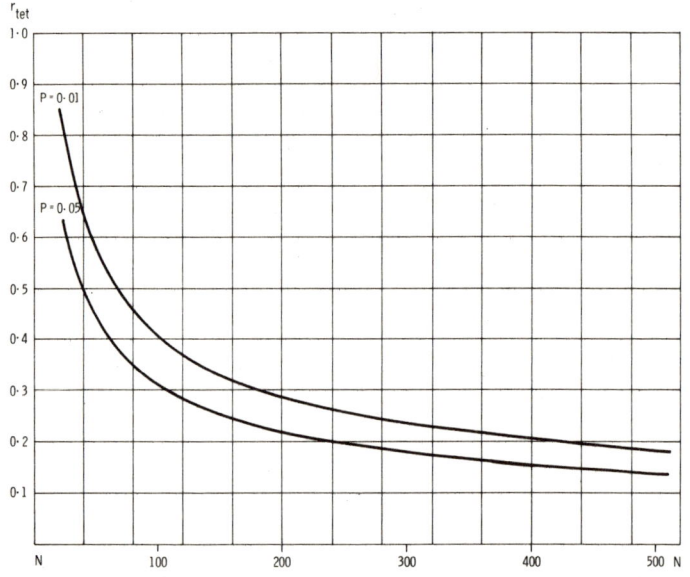

Fig. 8. Relationship between number of candidates and the value of r_{tet} required to reach significance at the 5 per cent and 1 per cent levels.

The standard error of a tetrachoric r of zero is given by the expression

$$\sigma r_{tet} = \frac{\sqrt{pp'qq'}}{yy'\sqrt{N}}$$

where p is the *proportion* of candidates in the upper (or lower) half for total score and q is 1 - p, while p' and q' are the corresponding proportions for question score, y and y' are the ordinates of the normal distribution for the observed values of p and p', and N is the number of candidates. The construction of the fourfold table (p.75) for the calculation of ad/bc will have the effect of making p and p' equal to 0.5 or very near it

Table for estimating the tetrachoric correlation coefficient from ad/bc

r_{tet}	ad/bc	r_{tet}	ad/bc	r_{tet}	ad/bc
.00	0-1.00	.35	2.49-2.55	.70	8.50-8.90
.01	1.01-1.03	.36	2.56-2.63	.71	8.91-9.35
.02	1.04-1.06	.37	2.64-2.71	.72	9.36-9.82
.03	1.07-1.08	.38	2.72-2.79	.73	9.83-10.33
.04	1.09-1.11	.39	2.80-2.87	.74	10.34-10.90
.05	1.12-1.14	.40	2.88-2.96	.75	10.91-11.51
.06	1.15-1.17	.41	2.97-3.05	.76	11.52-12.16
.07	1.18-1.20	.42	3.06-3.14	.77	12.17-12.89
.08	1.21-1.23	.43	3.15-3.24	.78	12.90-13.70
.09	1.24-1.27	.44	3.25-3.34	.79	13.71-14.58
.10	1.28-1.30	.45	3.35-3.45	.80	14.59-15.57
.11	1.31-1.33	.46	3.46-3.56	.81	15.58-16.65
.12	1.34-1.37	.47	3.57-3.68	.82	16.66-17.88
.13	1.38-1.40	.48	3.69-3.80	.83	17.89-19.28
.14	1.41-1.44	.49	3.81-3.92	.84	19.29-20.85
.15	1.45-1.48	.50	3.93-4.06	.85	20.86-22.68
.16	1.49-1.52	.51	4.07-4.20	.86	22.69-24.76
.17	1.53-1.56	.52	4.21-4.34	.87	24.77-27.22
.18	1.57-1.60	.53	4.35-4.49	.88	27.23-30.09
.19	1.61-1.64	.54	4.50-4.66	.89	30.10-33.60
.20	1.65-1.69	.55	4.67-4.82	.90	33.61-37.79
.21	1.70-1.73	.56	4.83-4.99	.91	37.80-43.06
.22	1.74-1.78	.57	5.00-5.18	.92	43.07-49.83
.23	1.79-1.83	.58	5.19-5.38	.93	49.84-58.79
.24	1.84-1.88	.59	5.39-5.59	.94	58.80-70.95
.25	1.89-1.93	.60	5.60-5.80	.95	70.96-89.01
.26	1.94-1.98	.61	5.81-6.03	.96	89.02-117.54
.27	1.99-2.04	.62	6.04-6.28	.97	117.55-169.67
.28	2.05-2.10	.63	6.29-6.54	.98	169.68-293.12
.29	2.11-2.15	.64	6.55-6.81	.99	293.13-923.97
.30	2.16-2.22	.65	6.82-7.10	1.00	923.98 —
.31	2.23-2.28	.66	7.11-7.42		
.32	2.29-2.34	.67	7.43-7.75		
.33	2.35-2.41	.68	7.76-8.11		
.34	2.42-2.48	.69	8.12-8.49		

Reproduced by permission from Davidoff and Goheen (1953). For further information on the accuracy of the statistical estimate obtained by this method, see Davidoff (1954).

and for these conditions the standard error is $1.57/\sqrt{N}$. A tetrachoric r which is 1.96 times the standard error is significant at the 5 per cent level and one which is 2.58 times the standard error is significant at the 1 per cent level. These relations are expressed in the graph (Fig. 8). If the number of candidates is entered on the horizontal scale, the values of r_{tet} required to attain significance at the 5 per cent and 1 per cent levels can be read off on the vertical scale. Thus, for the 50 candidates in the example quoted on page 75, values of 0.44 and 0.57 respectively are required. The observed figure, +0.81, is undoubtedly significant at the 1 per cent level. However, reference to Figure 7 (Appendix A) which indicates the levels required for Pearson's r, shows that for the same number of candidates the values needed are much lower, 0.28 and 0.36, and Figure 6 (p.73) shows that much the same levels are needed for the ϕ coefficient. This indicates the much lower reliability of the tetrachoric r, which is a consequence of the substantial discarding of information which its calculation involves.

REFERENCES

Davidoff, M.D. (1954) A note on a table for the rapid determination of the tetrachoric correlation coefficient. *Psychometrika*, 19.163.

Davidoff, M.D. and Goheen, H.W. (1953) A table for the rapid determination of the tetrachoric correlation coefficient. *Psychometrika*, 18, 118.

Appendix C:
Combining Correlation Coefficients

The standard procedure is to convert each r into Fisher's z coefficient, take the mean of the z's and convert this back to r. This can be done graphically with the aid of Figure 9, as follows:-

Enter r_1 on the vertical scale and r_2 on the horizontal scale. Find the point representing these co-ordinates and estimate its value on the diagonal scale by interpolation. For example, if r_1 is 0.60 and r_2 is 0.85 the combined value is approximately 0.75.

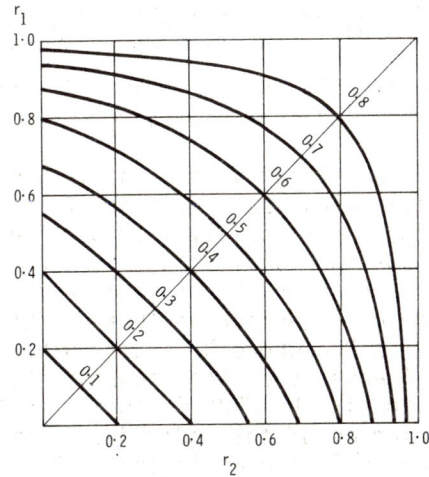

Fig. 9.   Graphical method for averaging two product-moment correlation coefficients.

Appendix D:
Tests for Internal Reliability

The KR20 formula for internal reliability is as follows:-

$$r_{tt} = \frac{N}{N-1}\left(\frac{\sigma_t^2 - \Sigma pq}{\sigma_t^2}\right)$$

where r_{tt} = internal reliability of the test
 N = number of items
 p = proportion of candidates making a correct response
 q = 1 - p
 Σpq = sum of (pq) values for all the items in the test
 σ_t^2 = variance of scores for the whole test.

This formula is applicable to items for which the score can be 1 or 0 but cannot be used for the +1, 0, -1 type of scoring system.

    The following reasoning may make the mathematical basis for this formula a little clearer. The score for any item must be in one of two categories - usually 1 or 0. The appropriate statistical model for such a situation is the binomial distribution and it can be shown that the variance of such a distribution (for example the number of 'heads' obtained when tossing a coin repeatedly) is Npq where N is the number of trials and p is the expected frequency of the occurrence expressed as a proportion of N. Σpq in the KR20 formula therefore represents the sum of the variances of the individual items. σ_t^2 is the variance of the scores in the whole test: the difference between this and the sum of variances of items is the sum of the co-variances. To define co-variance would be a lengthy business and it may simply be said here that the higher the proportion of total variance contributed by co-variance the greater is the internal consistency of the test. The expression inside the brackets can now be seen to mean, in effect, co-variance ÷ total variance, which is what is required. The factor N/(N-1) is a correction for length of test.

    Where the scoring scale is +1, 0, -1 the expression pq no longer represents the variance of a completion. Computer programs for scoring this kind of question do not usually print the variances or standard deviations of scores for individual completions, although provision for this could easily be made. It is unnecessary, however, when the program prints the variances or standard deviations of scores for entire items (made up of five completions) as is often the case. The variance of the item score is equal to the sum of the variances of its component completions scores, and hence the sum of the variances of all items gives the sum of the variances of all the completion scores. The KR20 formula adapted for use with +1, 0, -1 scoring thus takes the following form:-

$$r_{tt} = \frac{N}{N-1} \left(\frac{\sigma_t^2 - \Sigma(\sigma_i^2)}{\sigma_t^2} \right)$$

where N and σ_t^2 have the same meaning as in the KR20 formula and $\Sigma(\sigma_i^2)$ is the sum of the variances of the individual items. Note that N here is the number of *whole items* not of *completions*.

There is still some uncertainty as to the magnitude of r_{tt} which should be demanded if the internal reliability of a test is to be regarded as satisfactory. Most authorities would agree that figures of 0.8 and over are satisfactory, and anything over 0.9 is very good.

The general problem of reliability testing is discussed in detail by Cronbach (1957) and by Nuttall and Willmott (1972).

REFERENCES

Cronbach, L.J. (1957) Coefficient alpha and the internal structure of tests. *Psychometrika*, 16, 297.
Nuttall, D.L. and Willmott, A.S. (1972) *British Examinations*. London : National Foundation for Educational Research.

Appendix E:
Criteria for the Presentation of Projected Material

Candidates should be seated within an included angle of 30° each side of a centre-line to the screen. Moreover, no candidate should be seated closer to the screen than two image widths, nor further away than six image widths. In emergency situations the latter may be extended to seven or possibly eight image widths, but this is not to be recommended (Fig. 10). Stated in other terms, it is the ratio of the maximum width of the screen image to the distance from screen to the back row of seats (not the projector) that is important. This is sometimes referred to as the *Room Image Factor* and should not normally exceed 1:6. Equally, this factor should not fall outside these limits when more than one image is to be projected simultaneously.

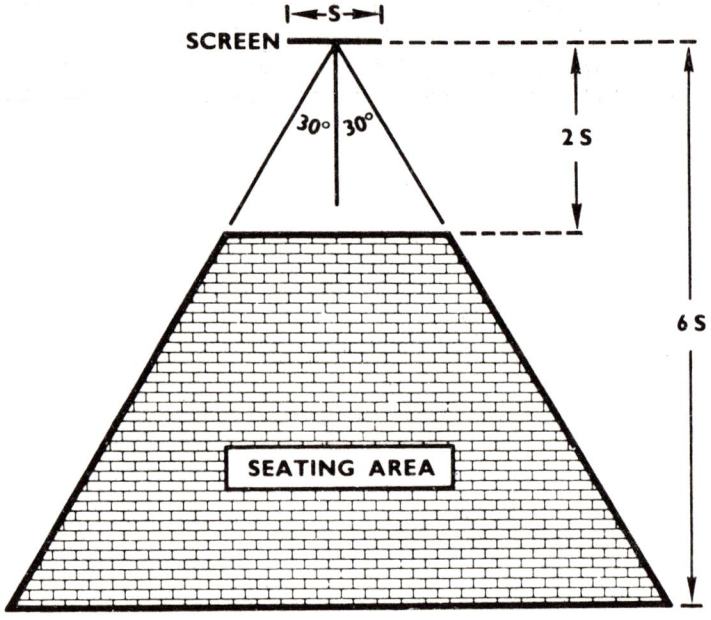

Fig. 10. Dimensions of the ideal lecture theatre, in terms of screen width.

Of the various screen surfaces available, a matt white finish is to be preferred for this type of exercise in which the observers are spread out over the maximum available seating area. Such a surface is generally easy to maintain and its condition should be checked annually. The British Standard for *screen brightness* in reasonable conditions of blackout is a minimum of *8 foot-lamberts* or *27 cd/m^2*. This should be adhered to as closely as possible, although it may be difficult to achieve in educational establishments. In no case should this figure fall below 4. Measurement is made of the reflected brightness from the screen with the projector focussed but without a slide in the gate; thus many adventitious factors such as the state of the screen surface and the condition of the projector are taken into account in this assessment. If screen brightness is found to be below standard, considerable improvement may be effected simply by attention to the following points:-

(a) Cleanliness of the screen
(b) Cleaning of any port or window through which the projection beam passes
(c) Cleaning projector lens(es) and condensers
(d) Checking voltage at projector
(e) Installing new projector lamp(s). This should be done as a routine to avert failure during an examination session
(f) Changing focal length of lens to reduce an over-large image.

No precise guide can be given regarding the permitted level of ambient room lighting for much depends on the size of the auditorium, the colour of its walls and the siting of the screen. Quite low levels suffice for writing answers after brief dark adaptation at the commencement of the session. Particular attention should be paid to the avoidance of any lighting pointing towards the observers and any spill of light on to the screen area is equally to be avoided. Deeply shrouded tungsten 'down-lighters' under dimmer control afford the best protection.

In the event of more than one projector being employed to reveal several views of a subject, it is imperative that the instruments are matched in every respect - in particular, lamp power, lens focal length and aperture. Since the brightness and size of each individual projected image must remain within the limits already prescribed, it follows that a much larger total screen area must be available for this technique.

For ease and quality of projection it is important that a uniform method of slide mounting is adopted and adhered to for all examination material; this avoids gross changes in focus between slides and facilitates indexing and storage. To aid the projectionist when the throw is great, as in a large hall, a pair of low-power opera glasses will assist in checking critical focus and the inclusion of an unobtrusive graticule in slide reproductions of x-ray films is of particular value in achieving sharp focus rapidly.

Various methods of timing the projection period of each slide will suggest themselves, but some form of visible as well as audible warning signal should be provided for projectionist and candidates alike. A total viewing period of two minutes for each single or multiple item with a preliminary warning of change at 90 seconds has been found satisfactory.

It is very important to have a clear numbering system for each slide or series of images. This can be achieved in a number of ways including the application of 'Letraset' or similar adhesive numbers to the image area of the slide direct, the use of an additional projector to cast an image of clear figures on a black ground on a free portion of the screen area, use of an overhead projector for the same purpose or provision of a suitably illuminated 'cricket score board'.

Peter Hansell

Index

Affective domain 5,6,7,10,39-48
    see also Attitudes
American Board Examinations 3
    Internal medicine 97
    Medical specialties 97
    Orthopaedic surgery 41,47
American College of Physicians 96
Analysis 67-79
Approach tendencies 39
Association for the Study of Medical Education 87
Attitudes, assessment of 6,7,39-48,89
Audio-visual techniques 24,27,85,86, 110-112
Audit, medical 96,97
Avoidance tendencies 39
Candidate evaluation form 41
Case histories
    see Problem-solving
Central Medical Examinations Service 27,86-88,95
Check lists 35,36,37,40,41
Clinical examination 1,6,7, 29-32,61,62
    undergraduate 34
    postgraduate 34
    design 35
    short cases 35
    long cases 35,36
    venue 86
Close-marking systems 8, 58,59,60,62
Cognitive domain 5,6,10,89
    testing in 11-28
    scoring in 50-60
College of Family Physicians of Canada 47
Comparison between schools 2,95

Computer based examinations 26,27,95,96
Computer capacity 83
Computer scoring and analysis 11,49,67,82,83
Confidence testing 53
Conjoint Board 2,16
Construct validity
    see Validity
Content validity
    see Validity
Continuing education 96,97
Continuous assessment
    see Progressive assessment
Core knowledge 2
Counter-marking 51-54
Correlation coefficients 69-76
    combination of 77,78,107
    product moment 69-71,102, 103,107
    point biserial 71,72
    phi 72-74
    tetrachoric 74-76, 104-106
Cost effectiveness 101
Criterion-referenced scoring 50,56,57,59,60,61,62,63
Criterion-related validity
    see Validity
Curricular objectives 4,91,92
Data interpretation 6,18,22,23, 24,92
Developing countries 34,100
Difficulty of questions 67,68
    Influence on discriminating power 71-73
Discriminating power 68-78
Distribution of marks 54,55,58, 60,62,63
Document readers 11,82
'Don't know' option 52,76,77
ECFMG 99,100

Essay questions 7,8,22,25,26,58,
   59,63
European Economic Community 98,
   99
Examiners 30,31,40,58,59,60,61,
   62,63
   briefing of 36
   effect on one another 60
   variability of 36,37
Factor analysis 45,46
Factual knowledge 5,6,12,14,16,
   17,18,36,91
Feedback 8,49,89
'Final' examination 2,7,33,34,89,
   90,92,95
Foreign medical graduates 34,99
Formative evaluation 43
   see also Progressive assessment
General Medical Council 1,95,99
Grading 49,58,62
Graduating examination
   see 'Final' examination
Hand-marking 22,83,85
'Hawks and doves' 36,37
Instructions to candidates 82
Interviewing skills 27,33,41,47
Kuder-Richardson formula 78,108,
   109
Laboratory skills
   see Practical examinations
Language 98,99
Memory clearing 90,91
Missing-link questions 24
Multiple choice questions 7,8,
   11-21,24,50-57,63,64,92
   answer sheets 11,15,82
   computer storage and
      retrieval 80,81,84,85
   construction of 18-21
   cueing 14,24
   distractors 12,13,16
   formats 12-18
   indexing 80,81,84
   limitations 21
   marker questions 56,81,84
   organisation 80-85
   overlapping 84
   scoring 50-55
   see also Analysis
      Discriminating power
      Reliability
      Validity
National Board of Medical
   Examiners 11,87,95,99
Objectives, definition of 4,
   5,18,21,49
Objectivity 8,9,10,11,25
Omnibus personality inventory
   45
Oral examination 1,7,27
   content 6
   organisation 86
   scoring 59,60,63
   unreliability 8
Paediatrics 32,34
Pass-mark 49,55-57
Patient-management problems
   26-27,57
Pattern recognition 21,22,
   24,85
   see also Audio-visual aids
Peer rating 50
Peer-referenced scoring 49,
   50,56,57,63
Percentile marks 64
Postgraduate examinations 3,
   34
Practical examinations 1,6,7,
   29,61,63,86
Predictive validity
   see Validity
Problem-oriented medical
records 92
Problem solving 5,6,9,14,18,
   21-23,26,91,96
Profile system 64-65
Progressive assessment 2,3,
   29,33,43,89-93,95
Projected material 24,85,86,
   110-112
Psychiatry 34,39,41
Psychomotor domain 5,6,10,27,
   29-38,61,62,89,92
Qualifying examination
   see 'Final' examination
Questionnaires 43-45,92,93
Ratings 40-42
Recertification 97,98
Reliability of tests 7,8,11,
   25,78
Relicensure 97

Review of examinations 83,84
Royal Australasian College of Surgeons 4
Royal Colleges of Physicians 3, 9,16
Royal Commission on Medical Education 86,88
Scales 44,45-47
    complexity 45
    Likert 46
    semantic differential 46
    thinking - introversion 45
Scaling of marks 51,55,57,63 64
Scoring 49-65
Self-assessment programmes 96
Simulation techniques 32,33,47
Short answer questions 25
Split-half reliability tests 78
Standard scores 55
Summative evaluation 43
    see also 'Final' examination
Syllabus 4
    see also Objectives
Taxonomy of objectives 5,6,7,12, 13,16,17,18,21,91

Test committees 70,80,81,82, 83,84,87
Three-option questions
    see 'don't know' option
Todd report
    see Royal Commission on Medical Education
TRAB 99,100
Translation of test material 99
Undergraduate examinations 1, 2,34
Universities:
    Birmingham 16
    Edinburgh 2
    Illinois 4
    Liverpool 2,16
    London 16
    Newcastle-upon-Tyne 2,16
USA, examinations in 3,12-16, 26
Validity 8,9,78,79
Viva voce examination
    see Oral examination
Video-taped interviews 27,34
Weighting of marks 53,54,57,60
Written papers 1,6,7,25,26,86